About the Author

Dr. Craig Brown was educated at Gordonstoun and followed in his father's footsteps to study medicine at Glasgow University. He did his GP training in Dumfries, and then in a mission hospital in South Africa – and found working with the Zulus fascinating, challenging all his perceptions of cultural norms. He has worked for the last 20 years in an NHS group practice and has maintained his lifelong interest in spirituality and holistic medical care. In 1996 he was appointed President of the National Federation of Spiritual Healers. He lives with his wife and four children in Sussex.

Optimum Healing

*A life-changing new approach
to achieving good health*

Dr. Craig Brown

RIDER
LONDON · SYDNEY · AUCKLAND · JOHANNESBURG

First published 1998

1 3 5 7 9 10 8 6 4 2

Copyright © Craig Brown 1998

Published in 1998 by Rider,
an imprint of Ebury Press
Random House, 20 Vauxhall Bridge Road, London SW1V 2SA
www.randomhouse.co.uk

Random House Australia (Pty) Limited
20 Alfred Street, Milsons Point, Sydney,
New South Wales 2061, Australia

Random House New Zealand Limited
18 Poland Road, Glenfield,
Auckland 10, New Zealand

Random House South Africa (Pty) Limited
Endulini, 5a Jubilee Road,
Parktown 2193, South Africa

Random House UK Limited Reg. No. 954009

Papers used by Rider are natural, recyclable products made from wood
grown in sustainable forests.

Printed by Mackays of Chatham Plc, Chatham, Kent

A CIP catalogue record for this book is available from the British Library

ISBN 0-7126-7107-2

This book gives non-specific, general advice and should not be relied on as
a substitute for proper medical consultation. The author and publisher
cannot accept responsibility for illness arising out of the failure to seek
medical advice from a doctor.

To my wife Elaine

Contents

Introduction

· ·

'Optimum healing is a journey: an exploration, an adventure. Difficulties are seen as challenges, and there is a search for meaning. The task on this journey is to release the negative and embrace the positive. The goal is peace and self-awareness.'

This book describes this journey. It is intended to help everyone achieve optimum healing for themselves, and has evolved from my experience as a doctor of integrating healing and spirituality into general medical care.

I have worked as a general practitioner for the last twenty years, and every day see a wide range of illness. I sometimes come across rare and serious diseases, but more often the common complaints such as backache, rashes, tiredness and sore throats. Yet each patient's illness is unique, due to their personality and life experience. I have found that with the steady advancement of modern technology and the use of more potent drugs people generally have an increasing expectation of cure. Illness is seen as an interruption in the frantic rush through life and they demand eradication of the symptoms to enable them to get back to work or attend an important social outing. The symptoms may indeed disappear with pills and ointments and even surgery, but unless the underlying cause of the illness is addressed, their health will deteriorate. It seems to me we have forgotten that the body is largely a self-healing organism and, when out of balance, there are warning signals to alert us to take remedial action. Sadly, in the majority of cases these signals are mainly ignored and not understood, not only by patients but by doctors too.

This book looks beyond the symptoms to discover what is behind your headache, nagging indigestion or tiredness. It is to help you understand why you are ill, and what illness may mean. This journey of evolving self-awareness does have a goal, and that goal is to find an inner peace. I took an important step myself on this journey some twelve years ago when I asked a spiritual healer to work in my practice. I had gradually, over the years, become aware that I never really got to the root of patients' problems. With my medical knowledge and skills I was able to relieve symptoms but the patients returned with other complaints. I learned that just listening with a sympathetic ear helped people through a crisis but then illness, often years later, seemed to date from that crisis. I knew that psychotherapy would help the more deep-seated and intractable problems, but to undertake that in a ten-minute consultation in general practice is an impossible task. Perhaps there was another way but at that time I did not know of one, although I lived in hope.

At those first meetings the healer and I exchanged our views about health and illness, and were able to discuss ideas and philosophies. I learned that healing is something very simple and natural that has been practised for thousands of years, and that any positive thought, word, or action can heal. For example when a child falls and injures themselves, a mother's first reaction is to cuddle and comfort the child. To smother it in love. The child quietens, the injury is attended to, and the self-healing begins. It is the mother's love that heals at all levels, emotionally, spiritually and mentally, and that helps repair the damage physically. Love acts at the spiritual level, and facilitates the healing of the body, mind and emotions. In medical care, prescribing drugs, performing surgery, giving advice can all be healing, as long as the intention behind the action is pure and loving. Similarly a smile, a touch or a kind word is healing. Healing is using the power of compassion as a real force in the universe.

A spiritual healer works with this same healing power or energy but in a deliberate way. He or she prepares for healing by first stilling themselves to find their inner core of peace. They then focus their attention on the highest source of peace and love in the universe that they can imagine. By consciously directing this power into themselves, and then through their hands, the healing energy is directed to the patient for their benefit. It can also be directed to the patient when they are not present, and then it is known as distant healing.

When healers say they are spiritual healers it is nothing to do with spirits as in ghosts and magic, but refers to the deepest level of our existence. It requires commitment and experience to become a practising healer and that is why most healing organisations have training programmes and supervision over several years. (I trained to become a healer myself and had the honour, in 1997, of being asked to be the President of the National Federation of Spiritual Healers in Great Britain.)

But to return to twelve years ago: after learning about healing I began to refer patients to the healer who joined us in the practice. They soon reported back the benefits they had received from this healing. There were no miracle cures but many said they felt better, calmer and more at peace with themselves. This was interesting in itself as the changes were not only in their symptoms but how they felt in themselves. I read up on the published research on healing and discovered its beneficial effects in all kinds of experiments involving plants, animals and humans too. I carried out some research in my own practice, and showed that healing certainly improved the patients' quality of life, and in many cases relieved symptoms.

Wanting to learn more, I invited the healer to sit in on my surgeries. I was interested in applying the ideas behind healing myself, and using them to find a practical way of getting to the root of patients' problems. In other words heal them. After each consultation in the morning surgery, as well as making the usual medical diagnosis, we would discuss what we felt to be the root problem of the patient we had just seen. This we called the spiritual diagnosis. At first it was a light-hearted game, but we soon realised it often seemed to hit the mark. Over a two-week period I begun to record the spiritual diagnosis as well as the usual medical diagnosis of patients attending my surgery. There was no formal method but it was a combination of deduction and intuition, which the healer and I would check out with each other. Over this two-week period I recorded 240 spiritual diagnoses. Examples would be: jealousy, dependency, helplessness, shame and resentment.

Altogether there were over fifty different words on this list of spiritual diagnoses. However, many seemed to be variations of the same basic attributes: irritation, annoyance, aggravation and hate are all variations of anger. From grouping other similar descriptions I was able to reduce the fifty to ten. So I now had ten separate causes as the root of all illness. These consisted of two main groups: the five negative attributes of anger, depression, guilt, attachment and worry; and the five fears of illness, accidents, change, old age and death. It was extraordinary to think that all illness could be reduced to these ten causes. However if you consider each one, they are pretty major problems in their own right.

Having identified the root causes was only the beginning because what I then needed was a spiritual treatment to tackle each one. This is the task of this book, to be a self-help guide to understanding illness and finding peace.

At first glance one may think that some of these diagnoses are more emotions and not spiritual at all. For example anger is normally thought of as an emotion. At the level of immediate experience it is an emotion which is very real when we are angry. However when anger is present without the person actually experiencing the anger at the time, it is then at a deeper level which could be called spiritual. I would say that an emotion is when you are experiencing the feeling in the present, where the deeper spiritual level may not be conscious.

One can seen the difficulty when trying to describe something like the consciousness of the mind, and then trying to divide it into compartments. The classification I have used is simply to create a framework from which to understand spiritual problems in a medical setting. They are not meant to be immovable pillars of dogma. The approach I describe throughout this book is what I have found to be helpful and is simply one way of approaching spirituality in medicine, which I have called optimum healing. I hope the ideas and practical suggestions are helpful to the reader on his or her own path through life.

Getting in touch with this spiritual core in oneself is the key to healing. Illness can no longer be described as the elimination of symptoms, the temporary patching up or dampening down. It is getting to the root and tackling the problem there that is important. The very process of casting off negative attributes and facing fear as a challenge is therapeutic. However, reaching this spiritual core is not the sole aim but, rather, the aim of optimum healing is to find peace and become more spiritually aware. The doctor's job in this self-healing process is to act as a facilitator.

Principles of optimum healing

- **To let go of the negative**
  Anger, depression, attachment, worry and guilt are the negative attributes at the root of illness.
- **To see problems as challenges**
  Illness, change, accidents, old age and death are challenges, and useful lessons in themselves.
- **To heal rather than cure**
  Cure is the elimination of problems. Healing is finding wholeness and harmony.
- **To look for meaning**
  Every event in our life has a purpose.
- **To seek peace**
  The aim of optimum healing is peacefulness.
- **To develop spiritual awareness**
  We are all spiritual beings who have bodies, a mind and emotions. Being alive is an opportunity for advancing on our soul's journey.
- **To embrace positive spiritual qualities**
  Positive qualities are the foundation of all humane living.

These principles may be new concepts to you and it can take time to begin to grasp how they are different from the way we normally view the world. This is a new approach to health but one I think, as you read this book, you will find rings true. Below I discuss these principles of optimum healing in some detail to give you a reference as you read on. I would advise you to read them once to give you a general foundation to optimum healing. The rest of the book develops the ideas with examples and practical exercises.

To let go of the negative

In the early work I did with the healer, when we made a spiritual diagnosis it was soon apparent that our natural state of health and happiness was being prevented by these negative attributes. What was apparent was that we needed to let go of these negative attributes as one of the primary tasks of optimum healing.

Illness itself has the purpose of drawing to our attention these negative attributes. It may not seem obvious at first but if we at least consider it to be a possibility we may begin to get a sense of what lies behind the illness. This is not easy but the task of the healing journey is to confront these shadow aspects of ourselves. They will never go away completely and, just as we feel we have overcome one, another will appear. However, as these negative aspects are released we will experience the benefits.

The understanding that, when we feel ill, there is a cause to our illness that goes much deeper than the physical and mental, is itself an important step in the healing process. The symptoms can be treated and helped at these levels but the illness is not ultimately released unless the spiritual level is also addressed. This book aims to help you in that process. As meaning is looked for, and spiritual awareness unfolds, the negative attributes will be released and the vision of peace opens up. However, just because I say 'spiritual' does not mean I am talking about mystical experiences; in fact the exercises suggested in the book are very normal and natural. The cases will illustrate how very ordinary people with everyday complaints in the setting of general practice are steered towards optimum healing.

Taking a broader view, it does not take too much imagination to realise that the negative attributes not only hinder personal development but also cause suffering and hinder development on a global scale. Famines are not caused by nature's failure to provide enough food, but by human greed and ambition. Wars are not caused by the other side, but by our own hate and intolerance projected on to the other. Our duty to humanity is not to go out there and save the world, but look inward and save ourselves.

To see problems as challenges

In the second section of this book I describe the five fears in the same way as the negative qualities, looking at common examples and trying to reach an understanding of these fears. I then look for meaning and discuss finding peace and developing spiritual awareness with the help of positive qualities.

The five fears are of illness, change, accidents, old age and death. The healing approach to them is that they have to be faced and understood, and to see all problems and difficulties as challenges, and to treat them as useful lessons. This requires a major attitude change. It is no longer a fight against these fearful opponents named death and illness, but a challenge to understand what is their meaning and relevance in our lives. Continuing to approach them with fear, and trying to battle to overcome them is not the healing way. There may be short-term victories but new fears will emerge and the suffering will go on.

To heal rather than cure

Defining health as the mere absence of disease is no longer adequate. Many people involved in medical care, including complementary therapists, still consider the aim of their treatment is to eliminate symptoms. In other words, if the symptoms are cured, the patient will then enjoy full health. This is the main thrust of conventional modern medicine and, in my view, is no longer enough.

This is because there is more to health than being free of illness, since we can still feel decidedly unhealthy even though we do not have any specific illness. Indeed many people who attend their general practitioner do so without any specific illness, but will complain of tiredness or not feeling themselves. Ask yourself how it feels to be really well, or in optimum health. It may mean simply feeling good and having lots of energy. To others, it will be more to do with being content and having a purpose in their life. Thus a person confined to a wheelchair because of a disability can feel perfectly healthy, as a person who is dying can be at peace with themselves.

The emphasis on physical cure and longevity are unattainable goals. First, as we cure one physical ailment, another will inevitably appear unless we get to its root. Second, we cannot prolong life indefinitely and everyone must die eventually. Third, the attitude of focusing solely on the disease that is attacking the body does not allow for healing to begin.

Cancer treatment is an example where the body is seen as the battleground of a war fought against a feared enemy called cancer. With the optimum healing approach the suffering needs to be acknowledged by both the patient and doctor so they can, together, understand the illness for that patient and go on to seek meaning and purpose in the illness. Then a joint decision about any intervention can be made. Not only in cancer treatment but in every illness, what is urgently needed in health care today is a shift in thinking from curing to healing. That means bringing in the spiritual aspect. It is the awakening of our spiritual intelligence. This may seem quite a simple idea, but in today's medical care it is a major shift in thinking. What's more, this may be where the real advances in medicine will occur in the next century, not with improved technology but in practitioners working from a spiritual perspective.

To look for meaning

Science has brought great benefits to mankind in many fields, and nowhere more so than in medicine. We know a great deal about how each organ in the body works right down to a cellular level, and even the structure and function of molecules. We know a lot about diseases, their cause and treatments. Yet in our great quest for knowledge, and what is seen as the struggle to overcome disease, the meaning of illness has been neglected. Indeed, from the scientific point of view illness has no purpose at all. It is seen as an annoyance at the least and a very threat to our existence at worst. It has to be eliminated!

That viewpoint ignores the spiritual view which maintains there is more. Every event, every meeting, every illness has a purpose. We may not know immediately what that purpose is, but need to be open to discovering it rather than dismissing the unexplainable as chance or coincidence.

The individual wishing to achieve optimum health will see their life as having a pattern. It will be experienced as a growth, as unfolding. His or her life will have a sense of direction; perhaps to reach some kind of fulfilment. This attitude gives a sense of finding one's own destiny. It does not mean there is no suffering from illness, changes, accidents, old age or death. It means accepting there simply is suffering. That is the way things are. It is the reality of being alive in this world. This is not a negative view, because this acceptance allows us to search for meaning in each experience. It makes life interesting and exciting.

This is not just a philosophical concept that has no application in practical terms, because this search for meaning in illness may itself be the very key that opens the door to optimum health. It has been shown that members of self-help groups for cancer and heart disease who spend time talking about why they became ill not only have a better quality of life but actually survive longer. They explore what meaning their illness has for them and what part they contribute to the illness itself. Accepting responsibility for an illness gives one the best chance to take action and bring about change. If you think your disease is caused by an outside agent, or it is fate, you may conclude that nothing can be done. On the other hand, if you consider that you may have contributed to the cause of the disease by changing something in yourself you are open to possibilities of recovery. Another dimension to self-help groups where problems are shared and there are no experts is that it is a way of empowering the individual.

WRITE A STORY OF YOUR LIFE

If you are serious in your endeavour to find meaning, reviewing your life is a start. Writing about your life can be quite a big task, but perhaps you can at first write a short résumé. Start at the beginning and tell it as a story. Such an exercise will help you to see how you have travelled so far and help you discover any patterns. Do not worry if you do not immediately find some kind of meaning. Most revelations do not come as blinding flashes, but often as little flickers of light. The important thing, as with any of the exercises in this book, is to do them and to be open to any thoughts that may occur.

Once you have written it ask yourself what kind of story it is: a drama, an adventure or a farce? Is it a good story, and who is the star, the director and the supporting cast? How does the story end? This kind of review or autobiography can be in any style you like; after all it is your story. It may begin to show you where you are in your life and begin to hint at its purpose.

Do you see your life as having a pattern?

Are situations repeating themselves, and needing a fresh way to resolve them? Unless life problems are treated as challenges that need creative solutions they will go on repeating themselves. In the film *Ground Hog Day*, the star wakes up each day on a festival day called Ground Hog Day. He gets a new chance each day to get it right, and the day goes on repeating itself until he does. Sometimes it seems as if our own lives are like this.

Did your illness start after a significant life event?

What was happening in your life at the time of the onset of the illness? This is an interesting question as it may give you a clue as to why you became ill. That then leads on to what your frame of mind and feelings were at that time. If these can be uncovered, it is a fertile area to explore as these attitudes are likely still to be present now.

Other questions.

When did you last feel well?

What do you think could be the cause of your illness?

How do you feel about the present situation?

Do you see any meaning to it?

How do you see things working out?

These questions are not to fill your mind with more analysis. Ask them then leave them. Make space for them to move freely in your mind, and slowly over a period of time an answer will emerge.

To seek peace

There is a new vision for medical care. We will no longer view ourselves as physical beings fighting against illness and trying to extend our lives but as spiritual beings living in each moment, letting go of negative attributes, seeing adversity as a challenge, searching for meaning and striving towards peace. The outcome of medical treatments will not be measured solely by the relief of symptoms, or by living longer, but whether patients have moved towards a more peaceful state.

If we think of the care of the dying, successful care is when the patient dies peacefully. It is not a failure to die. Similarly, in cancer care, there needs to be a move towards quality of survival, and not just quantity. This approach should be central to all medical care, and not an extra.

What is, and where is this peace that we all yearn for? Peace in the world, peace at work, peace in our relationships? This peace of mind is not found 'out there'. It is an inner journey, a journey of optimum healing to reach that place of complete stillness at the centre of our true nature. This task of looking inward is not an escape from the world into ourselves, but a means of being more deeply involved and making a creative contribution. When we reach that total calmness we can hear the whisper of ideas, offering solutions to our problems, often bringing a sparkle to a dark place. The simple fact is that, to rediscover this peace, we have to change: change our thoughts and attitudes, and change the very way we live and act.

So often patients who consult me in the surgery need to be reminded to find some quiet time to themselves. It is all too easy to go through the day without a break or even go for weeks without a day off. As a result they become tired and irritable, and illness will develop. Everyone needs to plan in to their daily schedule some breaks so they can remind themselves of how it feels to be peaceful. Five to ten minutes of quiet is a way of bringing ourselves back into touch with our self. It is common sense for anyone at work, as it recharges our batteries and helps us to carry on more efficiently and effectively. It gives us space to view the bigger picture, to enable us to shape decisions about the changes we need to make. I myself try to remember to have a few quiet minutes before seeing patients each morning so I can begin with a sense of peace and give a feeling of peace to the patients who consult me on that day. On the days I remember to do so I find I am much more relaxed and the whole day goes more smoothly. I am sure the patients benefit too.

To develop spiritual awareness

Besides finding peace, the awakening of one's spiritual nature is the other goal of optimum healing. Perhaps they are the same!

The whole subject of consciousness and spiritual awareness is a lifetime study and what I have attempted to do is to make this as simple as possible, so we can begin to move on the path of optimum healing. If we can get in touch with this deeper level of our being and make changes we are on the right track.

So, to start, I offer some explanations of the terms used in this book: ego consciousness, soul consciousness, God consciousness, collective consciousness.

In normal waking life our awareness, or conscious focus, is mainly on the I part of ourselves. *I* want, *I* feel, *I* think, *I* experience. It is how we see ourselves and to some extent how others see us: 'I am intelligent, strong, shy, an untidy person.' This can be called ego awareness, or *ego consciousness*. To function outwardly in the world as a personality we need that kind of awareness, but not exclusively, as such labelling tends to limit our ability to change.

If we focus inwardly at a deeper level of our being we can get a sense of something other than body, mind and emotions. This is what I will refer to as *soul consciousness*. The core of our being is peaceful and a source of wisdom, giving a glimpse of the divine within.

The experience of the divine without (or supreme soul) is what I have called *God consciousness*. Finally at that same level of greater awareness, we may begin to experience being part of, and connected to, everyone and everything. This, I have called *collective consciousness*. We may see the divine in others and, although we appreciate their uniqueness, realise they are essentially the same as us. That understanding is the key to personal and global harmony.

Underpinning the four aspects of spiritual awareness are the four statements:

Ego consciousness	We each use a personality to relate to the outer world.
Soul consciousness	We are immortal souls with eternal spirits.
God consciousness	The supreme soul is God.
Collective consciousness	We are each part of a whole, and interdependent.

The discussion of what is consciousness and mind could take a whole book in itself but, as my main aim is to give practical help in achieving better health for those who wish to pursue the path of optimum healing, I have tried to draw out the elements most important for this purpose.

SOUL CONSCIOUSNESS

As I have already discussed, the reality is that we are more than mind, body and emotion. We are spiritual beings and at our centre is the soul. We are all souls living in a body, we have a mind, and we experience emotions. The soul is the part that survives death, and so we can say it is immortal. It is uniquely you, with all your characteristics. However, these characteristics can develop and change throughout your lifetime. At the centre of the soul is the pure unalterable part, which is often called the divine spark. That is eternal.

GOD CONSCIOUSNESS

'God is the divine without.' That is a statement that has taken me years to say. I have struggled with the word God most of my life. I was brought up in the religion of Scottish Presbyterianism where God was seen as an authoritative male father figure. This view seemed to be reflected in the way the Church was organised, and how people worshipped. As I learned about history I was not too impressed by the Christian Churches' record of tolerance and compassion yet the simple message of Christ was appealing. I studied Gnosticism and Buddhism and many other religions and philosophies. I can only say that I gradually began to sense the presence of a caring, greater being - especially during meditation. This is my experience and everyone has their own beliefs but, more importantly, their own experience. This book has a non-denominational approach and is written to appeal to those of any religion or no religion. However, in a book which is about spirituality it is difficult not to use the word God. You may be more comfortable with the terms transcendent being, divine love, the source of peace, the essence, or supreme being. God is all these aspects, but please try to find the word that you feel most comfortable with. You may not have any belief or experience yourself of that aspect of awareness, but this book is still for you. We are all spiritual beings with our own and differing views of life.

My view is that as we are souls in a body, so God is the soul in the body of the universe. As we have a divine spirit at the centre of this soul, so God is the divine spirit of everything. As we are a being, so is God. In that sense we are made in the image of God. God is peace and love, and we are peace and love. Compared to God, we are a drop, and He is the ocean.

COLLECTIVE CONSCIOUSNESS

Even if we do not believe in the soul, life after death, and God, most people have some degree of awareness that life holds more than simply what is right in front of them. This is what I have called awareness at the collective level. It is appreciating a beautiful view, inspirational music, the stillness of a forest, the vastness of the ocean and the expanse of the sky. They are all spiritual experiences that do not depend on a belief in a soul or God. They often give a sense of wonder and awe. We appreciate that we are a small part of something very much bigger than ourselves.

Part of that collective awareness is the realisation that, in the vastness of time and space, the differences between other human beings are really quite small. Basically we are very much like everyone else. Not only are our bodies of the same basic nature but also our spiritual nature is similar. Integration of these concepts into our daily lives is the path to optimum health.

The other element of this collective realisation is how interdependent we all are on this planet. The health of an individual will affect the family, those he or she works with, and everyone with whom he or she comes in contact. In turn each person's health is affected by the environment, community, society, nation and whole world. I say this because if you do feel strongly about any of the global issues such as famine, poverty, or the environment the only way we can truly change them is for us first to change ourselves. If we can change, the world will change. It is a sacred undertaking to reconnect with our nature, and then express it. From that point of view optimum healing is not just an urgent personal issue but a global one.

To embrace positive spiritual qualities

What are the characteristics of a person on the path of optimum healing? What qualities or virtues would you expect them to have? What are the values on which they base their lives?

Developing this idea of spiritual values is a way of focusing on what is good about ourselves. It is not getting caught up in self-criticism, emotional feelings, past misdeeds or bodily needs. It is looking deeply at our own inner beauty. To help you develop this idea of spiritual qualities, think of someone you admire and whose life you feel to be exemplary. It could be a historical figure who was an inspiring leader, or a much quieter individual devoting his or her life to others. Then ask yourself which virtues they have that attract you.

The Buddhists describe six qualities or virtues they feel a person should have who aspires to lead a healthy life. These are: *patience, optimism, generosity, wisdom, discipline and stillness.*

In his letter to the Galations, Saint Paul says that the fruits of the spirit are *love, peace, joy, patience, kindness, goodness, gentleness and self-control.*

I would say any positive quality can contribute to optimum healing. To the qualities listed above one could add forgiveness, humility, simplicity, playfulness, humour and many more. It does seem that if a person acts, speaks and thinks positively, they gain benefit.

Which qualities do you have in the list below?

Patience	Kindness
Efficiency	Honesty
Generosity	Humility
Tolerance	Humour
Respect	Optimism
Consideration	Clarity
Purposefulness	Wisdom
Discipline	Joy
Co-operation	Flexibility
Trust	Care

One way of assessing which qualities or values you have is to give yourself a score out of ten for each value. Most people will see that they have scored something on each of the qualities. Which of course is the situation, as we all have these qualities in us, but they are not yet fully developed. Throughout the book I will be suggesting some specific qualities that can be used to help us on this journey of optimum healing, and looking at ways of integrating them to support us on this journey.

The optimum healing approach is one of integrating healing with modern medicine. It is understanding the negative attributes and challenges, and looking for meaning. Seeing as our goal not to cure, but to find peace and develop spiritually. And finally using positive qualities as our helpers on this journey.

PART ONE

Anger

Anger is something we have all experienced to a greater or lesser degree every day of our life. In that sense it is very normal and natural. However, it is how most people deal with anger that makes it a negative quality.

Anger can go very deep and include intolerance, resentment and hate. When expressed outwardly it upsets others by being abusive and destructive, often leading to violence. As a result we ourselves often suffer regret, and feel ashamed. If held inwardly and suppressed these powerful forces lead to illness, particularly chronic illness such as arthritis, skin conditions, and cancer.

Four facts about anger

Anger is contagious

Situations like the following highlight why anger *has* to be dealt with. Not only for our own sake, but because it can so readily affect others, spreading like a disease.

Jack Thompson was an elderly patient who came to the surgery to book an appointment to see a doctor. He was clearly angry when he arrived at the reception desk and when he couldn't get an immediate appointment he became quite abusive. The receptionist became indignant with his unreasonable behaviour, and so asked the Practice Manager to intervene. She was in the middle of doing the practice accounts and was annoyed at being disturbed. After speaking to Mr

Thompson she instructed him to sit in the waiting room while she, in turn, contacted me. Having just finished a busy surgery I was ready for a break. I was not pleased at having to fit in another patient, let alone one who was angry and had upset members of our practice staff. I don't know where Jack Thompson's anger started, but certainly in quite a short space of time it had spread through our medical centre.

Anger blocks communication

Have you noticed that when you get angry you shout and say things you do not really mean? You are not the least bit interested in what the other person has to say. If they do start to give an answer, it often just makes you more angry. Afterwards you can feel guilty about being angry, and even that can make you angry with yourself.

With **Mrs Bush,** the consultation started normally enough when she asked for some painkillers for her back. I asked her to expand on her symptoms and couldn't help but notice how irritable she was becoming. I knew something of her recent problems in that her mother had died five months earlier, and her husband had been off work for six months following an accident. She began to cry, and say how angry she was with the hospital for not diagnosing her mother's cancer early enough. I tried to show her that there might be a connection between her recent stress and her present symptoms. She became annoyed with the questioning, and said that I didn't understand anything, and could she just have some painkillers. She left the surgery very angry.

Afterwards I felt I had got it wrong but later learned that she had followed one of my suggestions and been to see a stress counsellor.

Anger can last

Anger as an emotion is often suppressed, and may be forgotten completely. However it is buried deep in the unconscious mind, festering away. It may be there for years, affecting our attitude and behaviour without us realising. Sometimes it comes to the surface and there is a chance to release the poison.

Mrs Ingles was seventy-eight years old and had been living on her own for the past eight years. On this occasion she was consulting me again about her old problem of vaginitis which had recently recurred. It seemed appropriate to take the opportunity to ask her again when it all began, and she replied that the cystitis had started after her husband had left her ten years previously. I examined her and told her I could find no serious condition. After a period of silence she said that she and her husband never really had much sex anyway. Then she quietly added he always went after younger girls. She began to tell me various stories about him, and I realised that he had sex with under-aged girls, and that probably included their own daughter. Mrs Ingles had received a letter to say he had died, and this letter brought back all her old bitterness and hurt from over fifty years ago. I prescribed some cream for her vaginitis which would clear her symptoms on the physical level. On the spiritual level I'm in no doubt that expressing some of her anger would also have helped.

Anger is often denied

Mrs Wilson was a woman who was unwilling to change her attitude, and it resulted in tragedy. She was sixty-five years old when she moved house to our village near the coast. Shortly after her move she began to develop arthritis. It was rheumatoid arthritis. She didn't respond well to the usual drugs, and was referred to a specialist at the nearby district hospital. Over the months she tried stronger drugs by injection, and resorted to increasing doses of steroids. The pain in her joints and her immobility progressed relentlessly. She rejected any suggestion that alternative therapies might help her, and dismissed any offers of assistance. As she deteriorated I asked what her feelings were about her predicament, and she said she felt very resentful. Her family had sent her off to the coast, out of the way, to retire. She was bitter and angry with them, and with society, at being condemned to this fate. She could not and would not let go of this resentment. Three years after the onset of symptoms she died of the side effects of steroids, a very unhappy person.

We often express a deeper spiritual problem in a physical way. A relationship is when two people are connected, and in the body the connection between two bones is a joint. Arthritis occurs when joints are inflamed. Resentment is repressed anger; resentment over a past relationship can cause arthritis. Now this may seem just a fanciful play on words. However, to begin to realise that deeply held attitudes are expressed in your body opens up possibilities. For instance, when one's attitude is changed, the illness itself may be changed. Not necessarily cured, but changed for the better – and that is a definition of healing.

Angela Gladstone was concerned that the episodes of her irregular fast heartbeat had become more frequent over the last year. She was now fifty years old and was worried she might be at risk from a heart attack. Examination of the heart did show that she was having some extra heartbeats. On all other counts she was physically fit. I did a heart tracing and blood tests to exclude any underlying cause. We talked about other factors that could be contributing to the symptoms. She agreed to check on her diet, particularly additives and coffee, to see if they made her symptoms worse. Also she would think about stress in her life, and tell me about it when she came for the results. The following week when I saw her all the results were normal. She said she had been trying to think of some current worries, but there was nothing in particular that came to mind. What she did note, however, was how she became very angry with men in certain situations. On reflection, she knew it to be the case but it often seemed to be completely out of proportion to the event. She had been thinking about this all week when it struck her that she was angry with her father. This was confusing as she was very close to her father, and had memories of him as a kind and gentle man. She also remembered that he bought 'girlie magazines' of which her mother strongly disapproved, and which he would secretly show Angela.

He talked to her about sex he had with other women. She was
ten years old at the time, and did not know what to make of this.
She felt loyalty to him, but knew it was wrong. She felt confused,
and became angry with him. She could not deal with the anger
at the time so shut it away in her mind. Now as an adult she still
had these strong angry feelings that made her heart race.

Such anger from the past, particularly if it occurred in childhood,
can persist for many decades, often showing itself as a physical
illness.

The meaning of anger

If the only results of anger are unhappiness and illness, one may
well ask what purpose it serves other than to disrupt! In fact, it is an
energy that we have to own. If expressed inappropriately it can be
a very negative quality, but creatively expressed it is positive.
Discussing three further facts about anger may help. These are that
anger is *your* anger, anger is energy and anger can be positive.

1 Anger is your anger

Central to discovering any meaning in anger is the understanding
that the anger we experience is not 'out there'. It is right here. It is
our own anger. We may feel that someone caused our anger, or
that someone deserves to be the victim of our anger, but the important point is that it is *our* anger, and it is *us* who have to deal with
it. This is a major shift in most people's understanding. The anger
they feel is not caused *by* someone; that person simply acts as a
trigger to ignite our own anger. If you think about it, there are situations which may infuriate you but not bother someone else, and
vice versa. It is not so much the situation that makes you angry, but
your response to that situation.

WHERE IS THE ANGER?

Next time you feel angry or irritated, think about how you
experience the anger. Does your heart race, do you shout, wave
your arms, become red in the face? Do not try to block it out by

saying to yourself that you should not show your anger, or feel guilty about being angry. It is better to feel it and experience it fully rather than deny it. Think about anger as a thing and note where it is in your body. Is it in your head, stomach or chest? How big is it, what shape and texture, and what colour is it? What is it like? Try to describe it in detail.

This exercise helps you to become more conscious of your anger, and stops you denying and repressing it into your unconscious where it can only fester and gain in power. Experience the anger fully first, then consider an appropriate way to express it.

HOW DO I EXPRESS IT?

You may already have your own ways of discharging the energy of anger. Many people find that physical exercise, such as a brisk walk or going for a run, seems to help. Often sports which tire you out are a way of releasing the inner anger although, sadly, we often see the negative, violent part expressed in sport as well. I know people who like to go down to the sea in a storm and have a good scream; others will shout as a train noisily passes. Some people vent their anger by thumping a pillow. All these are perfectly acceptable, although if someone triggers your anger it is not a good idea to think of them while being violent. Remember, thoughts have energy too, and have a power much greater than is generally accepted.

A twenty-six-year-old single mother consulted me because she was concerned about the outbursts of rage that occurred during the week before her periods. Her four-year-old daughter had been the target of her angry outbursts, and on several occasions she had hit her harder than she'd intended. Soon after, she felt extreme guilt and a fear that it could happen again. As a child, she had never been encouraged to express her emotions, and now for her own child's safety she held back her feelings. Various hormone preparations for premenstrual tension had been prescribed, and dietary changes had not helped.

We decided on a plan. The week before each period she would ask her own mother to look after the child for two hours each day; this would give her that time to herself to vent all her rage. She tried it – and once she got into her anger she could keep going for half an hour at a time. She destroyed several pillows by punching them so hard. On one occasion, in the middle of one of these sessions, she had an image of her ex-boyfriend, the father who had deserted their child. She found herself shouting at him, and bashing the pillows. Although, as I mentioned above, it is generally not a good idea to hold an image of a person while expressing anger, this is how she felt at the time. She began to look forward to these sessions of expressing her anger. After some weeks the rage lessened, and she was able to release the image of her ex-boyfriend and address the anger by using other methods. Meanwhile the relationship with her daughter had improved considerably. She'd needed first to express the anger emotionally; to get in touch with the deeper rage about her lost relationship with her ex-boyfriend. It took her a long time to let go of the anger that had been stored up for years.

PAINT A PICTURE

Painting is something most of us have not done since leaving school and we may feel we have no talent. But for this sort of painting you do not need painting skills, only a sense of fun! Get a large sheet of paper and lots of different paints, then try to paint your anger. Not the word anger, but the feeling. Paint your feeling of anger. Give yourself over to the task and let yourself go. This is a positive use of anger, and you may be surprised by your results. This exercise is more than just discharging the energy of anger; it is a way of channelling it creatively, and can prove quite satisfying. The same exercise can be done with other methods of creative expression, such as modelling with clay, and dancing.

2 Anger is energy

Of all the negative attributes, anger is the one that has the most energy. It ranges in intensity from a mild irritability, through annoyance, to a blinding rage. When we are angry we tend to become very het-up and full of energy. Some people may appear calm when they are angry, when inside they are burning up; others will shout and scream. Inevitably we all do and say things that we later regret. The energy of anger is very powerful, and can be quite destructive. If we quickly recognise it in ourselves the sensible thing to do is to try not to express the anger at the time; and if at all possible to withdraw from the situation to cool down. We can then at least assess the best way to deal with the current situation, and this will prevent us from saying and doing things for which we may be sorry later. However, this energy will only temporarily be contained, and needs to be dealt with soon before it festers away to cause illness. The end-of-day review is perhaps the best time to clear the negative attributes.

3 Anger can be positive

We have labelled anger as a negative quality because it leads to unhappiness, and generally this is true. But the energy of anger can ultimately have benefits, for it can lift us out of apathy and galvanise us into action. The passion we experience when moved by a just cause is an example of the positive energy of anger, as is having sympathy with the underdog or empathising with a tragic situation. Such passion is creative. It can inspire heroic action, or beautiful poetry. What I am suggesting is that anger becomes positive *if* it is directed in a positive direction, *and* is carried out in a positive way. For example, if you are disgusted with litter on your street and hold back your anger, the energy of your anger works in a negative way. But if you write to the authority responsible, or you even organise a 'keep tidy' group in your street, it begins to work positively. In addition, if it is done in a polite, helpful and co-operative way, still using the energy of the anger, the outcome will be more successful and powerful. *This is the process of transformation* and is a natural law. When a negative energy changes into a positive energy it gains in power at a spiritual level. The results are longer lasting, reach more people and have a greater strength. If you wish to prove this just try it out.

WRITE A LETTER
Think of an issue in your community that really makes you angry. Now try to compose a letter to the appropriate authority, but do so in the most caring and helpful way you can. Be polite and make positive, simple suggestions. Try not to be critical, only to express

your concern. If you wish to test the theory that anger can be positive then post your letter and see what happens! You can do the same by writing to a person who makes you feel angry.

DO I DESERVE THE ANGER?

If we find ourselves repeatedly in situations that make us angry, we need to ask ourselves why. Are we not learning from these experiences? Are we actually attracting the anger, and do we deserve it? Perhaps in the past we may have behaved in a way that triggers the anger in others.

The next time you are angry use the opportunity later to reflect why you became angry at that time. Asking such a question at a time when your intention is to change will nearly always produce positive answers. In other words, if your motivation is genuine you are more than halfway to solving the problem.

Who is my teacher?

It is often the case that the characteristics we dislike most in other people are the very things we don't accept are actually part of ourselves. If there is a particular person who makes you angry, examine the aspects of his or her character that annoy you and then honestly ask yourself if in any way you share these characteristics. Your first reaction will probably be to deny that you could possibly have such horrible attributes! This is quite normal. We tell ourselves we could never be like that, and think the faults belong to others. The part of ourselves that we deny is known as our shadow, as it clings on to us in the shadow of how we normally see ourselves. To think others have these qualities is known as projection, as we project our shadow on to them. For example, some people see all policemen as authoritative and aggressive. Others may consider all traffic wardens to be petty-minded and spiteful, teachers to be bossy, doctors to be arrogant, and so on; the list is endless. In reality they are normal people with families and difficulties like anyone else. But we all pre-judge them, and in so doing project our own negative attributes on to them.

Peacefulness

Anger is neither bad nor evil but it does cause us suffering and illness and can prevent us from finding inner peacefulness. Peacefulness is our natural state, and anger needs to be cleared out of the way to allow our real soul nature to shine through.

had a patient who used to attend with various stomach and chest pains, and every time I enquired into her symptoms she became angry. Often the consultation seemed to end in an angry mess, leaving her frustrated, and me with a feeling of helplessness, not knowing what went wrong. It was only when I discussed with her why she got angry with me that she said I reminded her of the way her father used to question her constantly about her activities as a teenager. She was seeing me as an authority figure in the same mould as her father. Once this discovery was made, her anger died down, future consultations were much easier, and I could get a glimpse of the person behind the angry cloud.

Acknowledging the anger, and then saying sorry if it has offended, is the simplest and most effective way of clearing it and bringing back a sense of peace. But it is not easy. Anger can make us feel energised to initiate action. It is an energy that gives us a feeling of power, and we can feel reluctant to let it go. Pride may prevent us from casting it off. But in those pursuing healing at a soul level, anger has no place, and, however difficult, it has to be released.

Finding peace in nature

If you are lucky enough, go to a favourite spot in a park or garden where you can sit and relax. If you are out in the open allow your mind to calm down, and listen to the sounds of nature. Observe the wonderful variation of colour. Breathe in the atmosphere. This is probably enough to bring you back into balance again. However for most people in a modern working situation it is not possible to visit a park or garden, but such a place can be created in the mind; it is just a matter of finding a quiet space in a room where you will not be disturbed. Remember to take the phone off the hook.

Imagine you are in a beautiful natural setting such as in a forest, or by the sea, or on a hillside. If you cannot remember such a favourite place, make it up. Even a couple of minutes thinking of being calm brings a sense of peace. If we have been angry it serves to remind us how much happier we are when we are peaceful.

Reflect on anger

We may want to be peaceful and think we are naturally calm when suddenly anger appears. It is useful to reflect on the anger when we are in a peaceful frame of mind, and ask such questions as:

> *'What is it that has upset my sense of peacefulness?'*
> *'Why am I angry now?'*
> *'Did someone provoke me, or was it contagious anger that has now made me angry?'*
> *'Am I still angry about something that happened yesterday, last week, or even last month?'*

This kind of reflection during calm times will help us to make balanced decisions about the situations that lead to such anger. We can then think of some of the ways we may deal with the anger now, or if such a situation were to arise again.

Create peace in your mind

Again find a quiet place, and sit so that you are relaxed. Now imagine you can see an empty white screen in front of you. Think about a recent incident that has annoyed you, or a particular person whom you find irritating and imagine it or them. You are detached; you are watching but you are separate from the scene. Just as with a video, you can play it back or stop it – and you can act as editor and alter any part at will.

Now conjure up an image of your favourite colour. Make a large cloud of that colour, which now surrounds and obscures the screen. The cloud carries the screen off into the distance, and with it, the trigger of your anger. Sit calmly for a few minutes and fill yourself with more of your colour. This is a useful exercise to do at the end of each day; you can put all your angry scenes on to your screen, and send them off out of your mind. If you do this regularly you will discover that such angry scenes become less frequent, and certainly less intense.

You can be endlessly creative with such images to overcome anger. For example, if the anger is furious and cold, think of it as a block of ice which slowly melts in the sun. If it is hot and raging see it as a fire which is extinguished by heavy rain. Certain colours are particularly beneficial. The greens and blues found in nature are the ones to incorporate in any images you make. Green creates calm and harmony. Blue is peaceful and healing.

For such exercises of the imagination to be helpful they must be done with complete sincerity. Time must be put aside so you can remain undisturbed and treat the whole exercise with seriousness. Take time to be properly relaxed and, working through the sequence at a respectful pace, try to see the images as they appear in order to bring in their true energy. These images do not come from 'out there', but from the very depths of your own unconscious; they are very powerful, and can be very healing.

Spiritual Awareness

As outlined in the introduction I have divided spiritual awareness into three levels to simplify the discussion. In reality there are no divisions or levels as they are all one. Such paradoxes often arise as you explore spirituality. When you feel you have grasped the meaning of something, either its structure or its sense, the opposite may well have equal meaning. This is the paradox. It is best just to accept it, and not concern yourself with the philosophical details, unless that is of particular interest to you.

Soul consciousness

One minute we can feel calm and relaxed, and the next we can be all fired up with anger. And equally quickly we can calm down. This shows us that anger is not permanent. Not only that, but it is not part of the essential soul nature we are born with. The soul is immortal. It existed before entering the body, and will continue to exist after the body dies. We need to learn to focus less on our anger, and become aware of the spiritual level of our being. That way, the anger becomes less a part of our personality.

However, very few of us experience ourselves at such a level most of the time. To do so we must set time aside each day to get to know this part of our being. When you begin to experience anger, the trick is rather than focus on the anger tune into the soul conscious-ness level of your being, just to remind yourself who you truly are. At first it is not easy; it requires time and effort trying to break the habit of a lifetime! But remember anything worth while is not going to be easy. We are, after all, striving towards a high ideal.

God consciousness

Mrs Johnson's complaint was heartburn, and it had started shortly after her husband's death. I knew her to be a regular churchgoer, and she often spoke of the charities she worked for. She talked some more, and went on to say how she had felt her husband had died sooner than expected. She was angry with God for taking him away.

It is not an uncommon experience to feel angry after a loved one dies, and to direct the sense of injustice at God. Such negative feel-ings are a challenge to ask such questions as: What is God like? Is He or She the sort of being who is going to subject us to unneces-sary suffering? What is our relationship to this being? Is it a father-daughter relationship, or mother-daughter relationship? Do we see Him/Her as a friend, trusted companion, compassionate mentor, or all of these?

I asked Mrs Johnson this sort of question and initially they unset-tled her so much that she consulted her parish priest for support. He was able to help her to face up to some of these difficult issues, and in so doing she was expanding and deepening her awareness of herself and God and was able eventually to let go of her anger towards Him.

A LETTER TO GOD

If you have been angry with God, write your anger down in the form of a letter, and expand on your feelings. It may be just a mild irritation concerning something you don't understand, or something more profound that deeply affects your faith. Often by forming a question and setting out the problem, the beginning of an answer will appear. The answer may not come immediately, or even next week, but it will be provided some time. We just have to listen. Maybe it will come in the stillness of the night, or even in the noise of a football crowd.

Collective consciousness

Anger arises in the individual, but can easily take hold of groups; or even whole nations. We only have to look at past wars and present conflicts in the world to see how anger gives rise to violence and warfare.

We may well ask, 'What can I do about such strife in other lands? I am only one in 7 billion people who live on the planet!' We cannot just dismiss it as having nothing to do with us, and hope it will not affect us personally. We do have a collective awareness which tells us that we are in some way connected to all living things on this planet. And this also means that each contribution is important. If you analyse it, the only real change we can make in the world is the change we make in ourselves. If we do wish to clear away some of the negativity in the world we need to start right here with ourselves. By solving even the smallest conflict within ourselves, in our own family, between friends, and at work we can begin to have an effect in our own communities. It is immensely satisfying to think that the effort we make to change ourselves acts as a model for all those around us, and that they in turn affect everyone they meet. Negative energy that has undergone change and become positive is very powerful. Such local changes, like a ripple in a pool, will inevitably spread. One small shift is the start of global change. We do have a duty to this planet, and all the people who live on it, and the best way we can bring about this change is for ourselves first to change.

The next example shows how a real concern for global problems and discussing ways in which they could be resolved can in turn help with personal issues.

Ann, a divorced mother, had recurrent headaches and was clearly angry about something. She readily admitted this and told me why. It was over access to their seven-year-old son. Her rage boiled up on mentioning her husband's name. Telephone conversations with him ended in angry exchanges, and she took every chance to criticise his part in the bitter battle.

On another occasion we had the opportunity to discuss some of the world's problems, especially conflict between different racial groups. She had some good ideas on how to resolve these international disputes, in which one side had to compromise first, and their differences at least be respected.

Suddenly she could see how the conflict we were discussing on an international level was very similar to her personal situation. She reluctantly began to admit her husband did have some good traits. She had never recognised this, let alone told him. She had found a good model with which to begin work on her own relationship. Next time her husband telephoned she was able to tell him for the first time how she appreciated his taking her son during her evenings at work. As the weeks went by they no longer needed lawyers, and began to work out a way in which they could share access to their son.

IMAGINE THE EARTH

Imagine the earth as a globe slowly revolving on its axis in outer space. As it turns you can identify the huge continents surrounded by the blue oceans. As you recognise the countries, think of all the conflicts you have read about occurring in these countries, and how those conflicts are the result of anger causing violence and wars. Now imagine a powerful golden light coming from outer space to surround the earth, which extinguishes all the anger to restore harmony.

As we begin to consider our own spiritual well-being, it inevitably increases our awareness of our responsibilities to the whole earth and every living creature. The spiritual disharmony brought about by negative attributes results in unhappiness and illness in the individual. It is also true on a global level, where the lack of spirituality results in the global problems of today.

Spiritual qualities for anger

You can improve your own spiritual health by developing positive qualities. These spiritual qualities are the building blocks, and the very foundations of healing mind, body and soul. It is the negative attributes that undermine our path to good health and cause illness. There are many positive qualities that can help to overcome anger, but I would choose foremost the positive qualities of tolerance and patience.

TOLERANCE

Tolerance is acceptance and flexibility;
And is listening with attention.
Tolerance is understanding that others are different;
It is meeting a stranger as a friend.
Tolerance is the beginning of love.

Every day our tolerance is tested. There are difficulties and misunderstandings in our families, with friends, and at school or at work. Everyone is different, and some may have personality traits that annoy us. We are often faced directly with the negative attributes of others, and anger can be the most difficult. That is when we need to practise tolerance.

Tolerance is not suffering a person or a situation so much that we feel like a martyr. Tolerance is the act of turning in to our true nature, and calling on the treasure house of our other spiritual qualities. Acceptance, understanding, co-operation, calmness, open-mindedness, accommodation and, most of all, love. When we draw on these qualities under the heading of tolerance it becomes powerful in transforming anger and the negative attributes of prejudice, ignorance, antagonism and suspicion which often accompany anger.

A **large Bangladeshi family** joined our practice list, and at first myself and the staff would complain about the smell of curry, their odd clothing, their poor English and their unusual demands. As we made an effort to understand their culture and get to know them individually the comments were more often on their beautiful saris and attractive children rather than the smell of curries. Tolerance helps to build relationships between people, and this forms the basis of peaceful coexistence.

PATIENCE

Patience is contentment,
And waiting until the time is right.
Patience is being disciplined,
It is living in the moment.
Patience is endless stillness.

It seems many people are in such a hurry to get somewhere that they get impatient if held up. That is when the anger starts. The spiritual quality of patience brings us back right into the here and now, and living in each moment. If you have planned to do something, you may find you cannot switch that expectation to appreciate what you have in the moment. Appreciate your immediate surroundings, or use the chance to turn your thoughts inward, and move towards peace. There is a kind of wonder to be seen in the mundane when we practise our connection to the positive spiritual qualities.

Integrating spiritual qualities

When you have identified a strong feeling of anger in yourself there are three steps to bring in the positive spiritual attributes. First, think of that quality; second, experience the quality, and, third, bring the quality into your actions.

When you are angry it helps first to think of the words 'tolerance' and 'patience' while the anger is seething away. Say them over in your mind and you will soon begin to experience them. Next, try to remember a situation in which you were tolerant and patient. This brings in the qualities at an emotional level. The third step, having become tolerant and patient yourself, is to demonstrate that by your actions. It can be difficult to integrate these qualities at the time of anger, and it is perhaps better to reflect later on the situation. Use the same basic method. When thinking about the words 'tolerance' and 'patience', think of other words with similar meaning. See 'tolerance' at the centre, and attach the other words such as 'understanding', 'openness', 'calmness', 'co-operation' and 'helpfulness'. This kind of mental exercise helps to expand the breadth of your understanding of tolerance's qualities, while remaining focused on the quality itself. As you work with the word creatively it becomes an active exercise and that way it will become part of your being at a deeper level. Experience the qualities, then integrate them into action.

Remember the case of Jack Thompson who was angry with the receptionist that I mentioned earlier? His anger had been quite contagious. The Practice Manager had asked him to wait in the waiting room while I went to sit quietly for ten minutes, which also gave him an opportunity to calm down. At first I looked at my own anger, and could see that I was tired and needed a break. I also felt indignant that he had upset me and our staff. But I tried to see it from Mr Thompson's point of view, looking at his anxiety about his illness, and the frustration of not getting an immediate appointment. Then I rehearsed the forthcoming consultation in which I would bring a quality of tolerance and patience into myself, and into the atmosphere of the room. When he eventually came into the consulting room he was still very angry. I let him express his concerns until he had finished. I explained some of the difficulties we have in accommodating everyone's needs into one particular system, then went on to discuss with him his illness and the significance of his results. He seemed satisfied, and at least calmer. I later learned from the receptionist that he had bought her some flowers as an apology. She felt a lot happier about the situation and so did the rest of the staff. It certainly made me feel better! So although anger is infectious, goodwill is equally infectious.

This demonstrates the third step: integrating qualities into your life by taking some action which embraces the quality. Everyday opportunities will arise to counter negative qualities with positive ones. There are plenty around in others, and lots of work to do on ourselves!

Affirmations

Write down on a piece of paper some of the qualities you would most like to have that may help you overcome anger, and then keep referring to it throughout the day. Keep it in your pocket or pin it up near you where you work. Examples other than tolerance and patience could be calmness, cheerfulness, generosity, acceptance and understanding.

can remember a very pretty girl who came to see me at the surgery in desperation as her complexion was ruined by acne. She had tried all sorts of creams, lotions, diets, even antibiotic tablets with little improvement. She said she was quite frustrated, and annoyed by any lack of progress in her treatment. The words she used and the inflammation of her skin suggested that she was angry about something. I suggested that she write 'I am tolerant of myself, and have a beautiful complexion,' and place this above the mirror where she washed every day, and say it out loud to herself every morning. Remarkably, within weeks her acne improved.

By first thinking of a positive quality, then experiencing it in herself, and finally doing something by writing it down and saying it out loud, that quality became part of her, and grew. Her own positive feelings towards herself neutralised the negative quality of her anger. The change started at a spiritual level and showed through at the physical level as the acne receded.

Preventing violence

To avoid potentially angry situations which could lead to violence, the key quality is alertness. Be alert to what is happening, both within yourself and around you. Also maintain an awareness of what could happen. This may seem obvious advice, but if you wish to avoid violent situations don't expose yourself to places in which you feel there may be violence. Some are unavoidable, for instance travelling home at night on a bus, on the Underground, or in a crowd at a sports meeting. These are situations we may not be able to avoid, or wish to avoid, but we can minimise the risk by being more alert. It is well known that black clothes and a sultry appearance attract violence. The same is true of people; it is better to avoid those who tend to be angry, and hence potentially violent. They themselves both attract and generate anger, and you may find yourself caught up in it. Taking simple precautions such as avoiding confrontations and backing off in arguments prevents their anger being expressed as violence. Try to be aware of other people's states of mind, and also how you are feeling yourself. There is some support for the observation that television and film violence can generate violence. The film produces an image that wasn't there before, and this needs to be resolved. If you are trying to pursue a peaceful path, violent television programmes or films are best avoided. You have a choice: you can simply switch off, leave the room, or do something else.

Protection

If you do happen to find yourself in potentially violent situations use this method of protection. Imagine there is a ball of light above your head. It is a pure light representing the power of love. It comes through your head down to the centre of your chest. It expands from there to fill your whole body and then moves outside yourself to form a sphere that surrounds and protects you. It can be a strong white light or a gold shell. Think of it as being impenetrable by negative qualities. You can use a symbol to seal the sphere such as a cross or a double circle. With practice it becomes easier, and more powerful.

On occasion I am called to the local police station to examine difficult and violent people held on remand in the police cells. I do feel anxious before visiting them in their small, dark cells. But I have found this simple technique to be very helpful; it is a protection for me and also calms the prisoners.

How to deal with anger

1 Understanding anger

Anger is contagious, it blocks communication, and it can last.

Anger is your anger, and is often denied.

Anger is energy, but it can be positive.

2 Questions to ask yourself

Were you angry at the time your illness started?

Where is the anger, and how do you express it?

Do I deserve the anger, and who is my teacher?

3 Things to do

Reflect on anger, and paint a picture of it.

Create peace in your mind.

Forgive yourself and others. Say you are sorry.

Be more soul-conscious and communicate with God.

Protect yourself, and use global anger to local benefit.

Embrace the qualities of tolerance and patience.

Depression

In the previous chapter I described the negative attribute of *anger* as outward and explosive. In contrast *depression* is inward and regressive. Anger stirs up energy; depression drains energy. The similarity is that both are contagious.

Understanding depression

Marion was a twenty-year-old nurse whom I was asked to see urgently by the concerned matron of a local nursing home, because she had found her crying helplessly in the changing room after work. When I saw Marion in the surgery she told me that over the previous six weeks she had become increasingly tired, was having difficulty sleeping, and was waking early in the morning. At work she had lost interest, was finding it difficult to concentrate, and felt very guilty about some minor mistakes that she had made with the patients. She felt that as she was more irritable than usual her friends no longer wanted to go out with her, and anyway that was pointless as none of the boys with whom they went out seemed interested in her. She sat hunched in the chair, speaking slowly in a monotonous tone, interrupted only by tears. She felt helpless and that life was pointless.

Marion was obviously depressed but in many cases this can be difficult to recognise. To help with this understanding I will describe most of the usual symptoms.

Mind In a depressed person, thinking tends to be slow and concentration is poor. Simple tasks like sewing or reading will be put down after just a few minutes, whereas usually one could concentrate for an hour or more. Thoughts themselves will tend to be pessimistic, focusing on past failures and present difficulties. Everything to the depressed seems pointless, and morbid thoughts are constantly repeated over and over again in agonising monotony. This experience of futility may lead them to turn to other sources of relief such as drugs and alcohol, which deep down they know to be destructive.

Body Headaches, neck tightness, tiredness, heavy limbs and lack of a sense of taste are some of the many symptoms. These physical symptoms are very real to the sufferer and often they will brood over them, thinking they suffer from some serious illness. Generally the body functions will slow down with a loss of appetite, and a tendency to be constipated. There is a poor sleep pattern, although getting off to sleep is not so much a problem as is waking up early in the morning.

Emotion In a depressive state the mood is low; typically, it is a feeling of heaviness, lassitude and weariness. This feeling varies throughout the day. It is much worse first thing in the morning and tends to get slightly better as the day progresses. But the mood goes downhill again in the evening. People who are depressed emotionally are 'flat', slow to respond to any exciting, interesting or, indeed, humorous situations. The tears of depression are often helpless, empty tears.

Spirit The depressed person is basically unhappy. Life has no meaning and lacks purpose; there is a sense of hopelessness and helplessness. The person does not feel fully alive. The things that usually hold their interest – such as work, family, sport and hobbies – no longer have any attraction.

They have lost contact with the inner self; not only who they are, but where they have come from, and where they are going. The sense of being connected to all things, being part of something greater than themselves, the sense of joy and wonder is lost and forgotten.

A common symptom at all levels of depression is the lack of vitality. At one end of the scale this shows itself as weariness; at the other, a deep despair. The depressed person feels depleted and lacks energy; lacks enthusiasm and has a pessimistic view of the future.

The energy levels can change throughout the month. Most women will tell you that theirs is at its highest just after a menstrual period and at its lowest just before. Their emotional state is also at a high and low during these corresponding times of the month. I am sure most women are aware of this fact, but if you do suffer from premenstrual tension it is a useful tip to avoid undertaking important decisions – or extra work – in the week before your period is due. What is generally less appreciated is that men's moods and vitality levels alter in a similar state which bears a direct relationship to the menstrual cycle of the women in their lives!

A further spiritual feature in depression is a lack of self-love. It is difficult to know which comes first: the depression, or the poor self-esteem. But this certainly is a prominent part of depression. There is a feeling of blame for past mistakes, including their own current depression which adds to the feeling of unworthiness.

An exercise that we did in the introduction reminds us of our own qualities, when we gave ourselves a score of 1–10 against a list of positive spiritual qualities.

Most people will have given a score against each quality which demonstrates that we all have these qualities, each to different degrees of development. When you are feeling low remind yourself over and again what your best three qualities are that go to make you the special person you are.

Even when we understand the symptoms and everyone does their best to help, the depressed person often remains closed off. Such despair is the lowest point of depression. It is as though we have been placed in an empty landscape, or put down a hole in the darkest prison. We feel we are all alone, with no help. The experience is filled with fear. It is terrifying. You may have experienced that feeling of despair after the death of a friend or when a catastrophe has occurred, such as the house burning down and all your treasured possessions lost. A loved one may betray you, shattering your confidence, or suddenly you are made redundant after giving your life to a particular career. You may be immobilised by illness, or let down by a political or religious ideal. The experience is one of utter abandonment and helplessness. The sufferer feels he or she will be stuck in this situation for ever. There is complete inertia.

However, things are always in a state of change, and even despair is not fixed. The future, no matter how bleak and forbidding it may appear, cannot be as bad as this unfamiliar and frightening experience at the depth of despair. The only solution is to explore a healing approach to this all too common problem.

The search for meaning

We begin to find some meaning in depression if we observe the pattern of nature. Here, change is the natural order of things. The annual cycle of the year has its high point of abundance in the summer, and its low point of stagnation in the winter. Summer moves inexorably towards winter and winter towards summer. Winter is a time for rest and recuperation, and depression may serve a similar purpose in our own life cycle when we need time for introspection.

Andrew **was a** forty-eight-year-old businessman who hadn't visited the surgery for five years and came complaining of tiredness, and difficulty in concentrating at work. He found that he lacked his usual vitality and particularly had no enthusiasm for his main interests, which were sailing and cycling. It turned out that he'd had only one day off work over the past nine months, and had been doing overtime on projects up to eighteen hours a day without a break. Even he seemed surprised when he realised how hard he had been working. The physical and mental fatigue had begun to wear him down, and was now showing itself as a depression. His thinking was slow, self-centred, and self-critical.

This slowing down generally may itself be part of the meaning of depression. Andrew's life had been going too fast for too long. His illness was telling him to slow down. Starting his treatment was straightforward; what he needed was time off work. He could use that time to take stock, and to look carefully at his life.

It is important to be aware that our own lives are made up of changing experiences: joyful events, disappointments, happy and unhappy times, positive and negative experiences. They are all transient. If we can learn to deal with the minor ups and downs of life, it certainly will put us in good stead to deal with any major problems when we come across them.

As all experiences come and go, and none last, we can learn not to identify too much with each experience and remain focused on our inner, peaceful nature. This is true of positive experiences as well. I am not advocating that we should deny things we enjoy, but that we should not become too attached to them. Even bad times get better.

Mary Hull sat in front of me saying her life was meaningless. She felt depressed, and no longer part of life. She felt disconnected from joy and, curiously, even from suffering. She was at a low ebb, and empty. She said she would have committed suicide but for the children. Slowly, over several consultations, we talked about her role of caring for her children, and she began to understand what an important and meaningful task it is to be a mother. She had rediscovered a purpose, and with that she could bear the inevitable hardships.

It is a struggle to find meaning when faced with despair and suicidal thoughts. One way in which Mary found meaning to her situation was to ask what was stopping her from taking her own life. In her case it was her children, but it could equally have been a dependent relative, a pet animal or feelings that there were still things to achieve in her life. It was the act of looking for meaning that shed a light into her darkness. That light grew until the depression lifted enough for her to feel able to address the causes of the depression itself.

But there is a point at which one cannot respond, even to the challenge of looking for a continued meaning. This is the pit of despair; the spiritual low point of depression. Not only is there a feeling of heaviness and darkness, but a complete sense of helplessness and hopelessness. Fortunately for most people this is only a temporary phenomenon, but if it persists it can lead to suicide.

Mrs Brown had only herself and her husband. They had no children or relatives, and enjoyed their own company. They did everything together: going for walks, gardening, shopping and household chores. They liked to go to the theatre, and were members of the local music club. Two years after retiring he had a heart attack and died. She was distraught at the time, and after several months was still in the depths of depression. Friendly neighbours tried to help out, but she could not and would not be consoled. After a serious suicide attempt the psychiatric services supported her as much as they could. She was on medication, and had bereavement counselling. Eighteen months following his death she threw herself down the stairs, and died two days later from her injuries.

If one can simply accept that what is wrong is a depression, the next step is to trust that things will begin to change for the better. It means beginning to believe that you *can* move through this dark and difficult time. There is actually no real alternative but to trust, to say to yourself repeatedly that your life is worth while. People who have been through the experience of complete despair will often later report that they found surrendering to this trust actually started them on the road to recovery. They made a reconnection with their own destiny and, looking back, felt stronger and richer for the experience.

It is difficult sometimes to find meaning in such suffering and perhaps the meaning of depression is to try to accept the ups and downs of the changes that occur naturally in life and trust one can go with that pattern.

Four ways to tackle depression

1 Think positively

Remember, we *do* have control of our thoughts, and thinking positively can be the first step on the road to recovery. I appreciate that it can be difficult to do this when one is depressed, but even a little positive thought can bring some light into a very dark place.

Liz Hawthorn was so exhausted that she collapsed one morning, shortly after getting up. When I visited her she sat on the bed, crying endlessly. Her tiredness and lack of vitality had been building up over weeks and, as it later turned out, had been caused by a whole host of personal issues. Despite her awareness of these issues she felt unable to share them with anyone, and so identified too strongly with all these negative aspects.

After Liz Hawthorn had told me all her problems I began to ask her about all the good things she had in her life. She had two lovely children, a roof over her head, a caring and understanding husband. She began to describe places she liked to visit, and the special friends who supported her. Just talking in such a positive way made her feel much better.

Life doesn't always go smoothly. We are not perfect, and we all make mistakes. But we shouldn't dwell on these too long as this will lead to a downward spiral of negative thinking. Liz's resultant depressive illness had forced her to rest. Only then was she able to reflect upon why she had sunk into such a condition. That reflection gave meaning to her depression, because the crisis then forced her to face the issue with a positive frame of mind. This is the key to escaping from a depression and it is also the most important step you can take to make your life happier.

Looking on the bright side can actually lessen the symptoms of illness, as the following story of an elderly lady's approach shows.

Seeing that her medical notes were quite thin, I took the opportunity to ask her the secret of her good health. She replied, 'I count my blessings, and whenever I get a pain or a problem I always think that there is someone much worse than me. That way, my suffering seems little compared with theirs. Soon afterwards the aches and pains go away.'

Looking on the bright side of a situation is an example worth following. Often when depressed one is preoccupied with one's own position. Consider the following questions:

Do I have clothes, shelter, food, and water?
Do I have freedom to express myself?
Do I have disabilities of body and limb?
Can I hear, feel, and taste?
Do I have a family and friends?
What possessions do I have that others don't?
Am I sane in mind?
Am I continent in body functions?

We may think our situation bad, but it could be a lot worse. Even when things are going badly it is better to fill our minds with positive thoughts rather than dwell on the negative. It is all about reminding ourselves how fortunate *we* are. As an exercise, referring to the above list, answer the questions. Then add to it the ways in which you are gifted, the skills you have, or your own particular blessings.

2 Make a recovery plan

Many patients I see say they work through their lunch hours, and do not even take a mid-morning or mid-afternoon break. They are too busy to stop. What they do not realise is that a short planned break will help them work more effectively. The break is not only for physical and mental rest, but also for spiritual renovation. This means actively relaxing, and using the time for reflection. Ask yourself where and when in your normal day you could fit in a break to relax.

It will not just happen. You have to plan. Make a decision where you can fit in these special times in your daily schedule. It may help to write down what you do in a day as a kind of activity diary: how much time taken travelling to and from work, how long working and how long for lunch and other breaks. Over a typical, twenty-four-hour period, how much time do you actually have to yourself? This does not mean time taken sitting down in front of a TV, but time when your mind can slow down; time when the thinking becomes calm and you can reflect on issues that have affected you over the day. Such time can be called true 'quality time'.

Getting out of the office for a walk helps to recharge the batteries, perhaps finding a quiet spot where you can sit undisturbed for five minutes. I know of a doctor who found that he always had fully booked appointments, so he began to make a ten-minute appointment with himself twice a day. That way he is not disturbed, and he uses the time for quiet meditation.

Do not feel guilty about having time off; try it. While all your colleagues are tiring from working long stretches, you'll find you will be full of energy. It is also important to have at least a half-day each week that is totally relaxing. Many people find strenuous physical exercise is a useful way of switching off, but equally walking, gardening or just sitting in the park can be revitalising. Each year there is a need to have at least one long break greater than ten days, and several days off every two to three months. So get out your calendar now and plan your time off. Planning is part of the depression prevention programme!

3 Draw your depression

Again, drawing can be a useful tool to get into a different mode of thinking. Do not worry about your painting skills! What matters more is that you can express your thoughts through drawing.

The subject to draw or paint is your depression. With an empty white sheet of paper in front of you ask:

'Where is my depression?'
'How does it look?'
'What colour, and what size is it?'

Try to draw this thing that feels so bad. The very act of trying to express it on paper is a healing exercise. Once the picture is complete, examine it.

Are there any areas that have interesting patterns? If so, begin to develop these patterns. If not, choose an area anyway, and develop it into anything you like. Moving out of a depression can be a very creative experience. This is another level in which the meaning of depression is locked up. If you can prise it open, it will undoubt-edly enrich your life.

Many artists, painters, musicians and writers produce their best work when they feel depressed, and use their art to explore the issues of life that are facing them. We can appreciate their art by identifying with what they are attempting to say through their work. Their efforts enrich our lives, and I am sure these efforts help the artists, too.

4 Follow the light

SAD stands for Seasonal Affective Disorder, the condition in which people become depressed in the winter months as a result of not having enough sunlight. I suppose to some extent we all recognise this, because we feel much brighter during the summer months and more withdrawn during the winter months when there is less sunlight. Natural light seems to affect our mood by cheering us up. On a winter's day there is nothing better than to get out and walk in the bright sunshine; it is common sense to get into the sunlight if we are feeling low.

Many exercises in visualisation also involve using light, as it is seen to be such a positive energy. This is a simple one to try. Sit comfortably in a quiet room, and experience the full darkness of your depression. Close your eyes and imagine, in the distance, a small bright light. It slowly moves towards you, illuminating the darkness, and shines upon you. You are moving on a path towards the light, and the light is moving towards you. As you come closer, it becomes brighter and stronger. It has the power not only to get rid of the darkness around you, but within you. All those dark, negative thoughts in your mind are washed away. You can feel the warmth and compassion of the light shining on you, caressing you like a blanket. As you walk on towards the light, you begin to feel better. You stand before it, allowing it to cleanse your whole body. Your organs, blood vessels and bones are all clean and clear. Imagine yourself to be washed by this light, and feel all the negative influences dissolve away. You feel whole and complete. As any negative thought enters your mind, it is immediately engulfed by the white light. Try to hold this experience for as long as you can. If feeling depressed do this for five to ten minutes several times a day.

Peacefulness

The method of finding peacefulness is outlined in the chapter on worry, but there are two exercises which are particularly useful for depression.

'How would I like things to be?'

Think about your future, the coming months and years. Don't think about your problems; how would you like the *future* to be? What do you value most in your life that would make you happy?

Give yourself permission to think about anything that would make your life more complete.

That **simple question** changed the life of Marion, the nurse I described earlier (on p. 40). She had had a difficult life, and had suffered from previous depressions which had not improved with therapies, including counselling and drugs. During the consultation her depression had affected me in such a negative way that I felt I had to bring in something positive to the situation.

I asked her that question: 'How would you like things to be?' Initially she was slow to respond, but then began to describe how she wished she could meet up with her sister again, have a boyfriend and feel well enough to continue with her nursing studies.

She left the surgery with just a glimmer of a smile. The following week, when I saw her to assess her progress, the first thing I noticed was a sparkle in her eye. Her sister had phoned, and they'd arranged a meeting. When they met, they really got on well. They both went off to visit their mother the next weekend. I saw her again four weeks later, and she was a changed girl. She was wearing bright clothes, was very cheerful and looking forward to starting her nursing career at the college. She mentioned that she had begun dating a boy she had met.

I had asked Marion to think of a positive future, and that one question had changed her thinking from a negative track to a positive one which set off a train of events. But I first had to change my own negative depressive feeling to a positive one before I could ask her the question. I had set a kind of template at a deeper level, which she then took on and was able to develop for herself. Such a simple question transformed her life. It also changed mine, as it showed me what an effect such a question can have. Now whenever I feel anyone is depressed, I always make a point of asking the question: 'How would you like things to be in the future?'

'A vision of a better world'

For this exercise find yourself a quiet place and allow yourself ten to fifteen minutes. Picture yourself in a country lane in the summer, going for a walk. It is warm and you feel relaxed, and are out to enjoy yourself. As you look around, you can see different shades of green in the trees and the grass and you notice the different colours of the flowers. You can even smell some of your favourite flowers. The noises of the countryside abound: birds are singing, bees are humming and the gentle wind rustles in the trees. As you walk along the path you come to a gate; and on this gate there is a notice. You move forward to read the notice, which says: 'Through this gate is a better world.' As you walk forward slowly to go through the gate, it gently opens and now, on the other side, you are in a better world. Immediately you experience its difference. You get a sense of what it is like to be in such a place. You look around to observe the countryside, the colours, the different shades and even the smells. You decide to walk on to explore this place further. Perhaps you see some buildings, and observe how perfect they look. You walk on and come across some people. How do they behave and how do they appear to you? Now take some time to sit and take in the atmosphere of being in such a place. When you are ready, get up to leave; walk back to the gate, remembering all the time how it feels to be in this better world and all the things you have observed. Walk through the gate to the country lane, then come back to the place where you are actually sitting.

When you open your eyes after such an exercise sit quietly for several minutes, and gently stretch yourself before getting up. I try to write down the images I have experienced, because this has the effect of making them more real and means I can go over them again later. Each time I do this exercise I always find something new. Its great strength is that it offers *your* vision of how you would like the world to be.

It is interesting that if you do this exercise in a group, many group members will have similar visions of a better world. The place usually has a sense of peacefulness and calmness. The countryside is green and bright, the people are friendly and caring. There is a great harmony between the buildings and the countryside. There is respect for all life; and everyone's basic needs of shelter, food and water are met. There is security and justice in the land.

When this exercise has been repeated in different countries and in different social groups throughout the world, it is immensely encouraging to realise that most people have a similar vision of a better world. This serves to show that there is a spiritual connection between all peoples on the planet. We all share the same basic values and are struggling for the same inner sense of peacefulness.

Spiritual awareness

Soul consciousness

To be aware that we exist at different levels of our being is an important step in overcoming depression in ourselves and others. We may feel depressed, but we are not the depression. We may behave in a depressed way, have morose thoughts and feel emotionally flat, but at the soul level that bright, pure light of our existence continues to shine. At the present time it may be difficult to see that light, but by focusing on the inner, bright light it will help to overcome depression.

At eighty-four Mr Ashby had a stroke from which he made a partial physical recovery. However it had affected some of his mental functions. Before the stroke he was a very precise and organised man; now he found difficulty with his memory and doing calculations. The result was that he became very irritable and depressed. By being optimistic, and reminding him of his inner qualities, over the months his wife and friends were able to lift that cloud of depression. They related to him at a soul level, and not to his physical disabilities, his mental impairment, or his mood swings.

God consciousness

It is difficult to believe in God when we have been brought up in a world of practical problems that are mainly resolved in an intellectual way. When meaning is looked for, and religion is turned to, it does not offer a satisfying answer for many. What then is one left to do and think?

Gordon told me about how near he was to suicide when he was depressed. One night he had walked down to the railway track and was ready to jump in front of the next train. As he waited, he challenged God to save him if he could. He waited and waited, but the train had been delayed; and when he looked into the sky he saw the faintest outline of the new moon. It seemed to offer hope; and he felt a rush of love pass through him. He walked away from the track. He was not a religious man, but from then on he always had the sense that some being was interested in him and would care for him.

If you do not believe in God, just imagine there is a beneficial being who wishes to support you through your problems; then see what happens. Does your life remain the same, or do you begin to feel that there is, indeed, someone helping you? You may say that this is wishful thinking; well, that is precisely what it is, and you will be surprised how many wishes are granted.

Collective consciousness

The next time you walk through a wood, by the sea, or in the countryside observe the beauty of the place and breathe in its atmosphere. Try not only to appreciate the detail, but also become part of it. This is the other aspect of being spiritually aware and when the connection is made it can heal at a deep level.

Jackie was a school teacher who, in the year following her retirement, became very depressed. She used to find herself walking aimlessly for hours in the hills. Her thoughts continually focused on how she could escape from this miserable existence. Then one evening, walking beside a lake, she saw the sun setting over the lake. It was the most beautiful sight she had ever seen, and she was surprised she had never noticed the beauty around her before. From then on when she went on her walks she thought less and less about the depressing aspects of her life and more about the beauty. She tells me just going into a wood, or standing on a hillside and breathing in the atmosphere makes her feel better.

It is the collective experience, being part of all of nature, that has this uplifting effect. We are also part of all humanity, and all beings are connected. This means that our attitude and our behaviour do have an influence on the way things are in the world. In a sense, we are a microcosm of the macrocosm, and we do matter. If we can overcome negative emotions such as depression, we are not only giving benefit to ourselves; we also serve as a role model to everyone with whom we come in contact; and in that way the world can be changed.

Spiritual qualities for depression: hope, enthusiasm and humour

Depression has no energy, so to help raise vitality we need to bring ourselves positive qualities that vibrate with energy and these three do just that.

Hope

Hope is being positive,
And is looking forward to a better world.
Hope brings light to darkness,
It is expecting the best of the future.
Hope is internal, external – and eternal.

It can prove difficult to be hopeful, even when we know it is right to try to be positive. Sometimes, however much we think about being positive it does not seem to work, as the next example shows.

> **was called late** one evening by a mother in tears because her son Gary had lost his temper and had smashed down a door. His mother was frightened, because he had been violent before. I saw the boy alone, and spent over an hour talking to him generally about his interests, plans for the future and things he had difficulty with. He seemed a fairly normal teenager; but when his mother came into the room his whole demeanour changed to that of a withdrawn, antagonistic youth. It was not that his mother was critical of him; the very opposite, she was 'smothering nice' to him. She had decided that the way to overcome his problem was always to think positively, but she could not be positive.

In any dialogue, we first have to recognise and acknowledge our own feelings about the relationship. Then we must acknowledge the other person's feelings. Only then can we bring into ourselves the necessary spiritual quality. In the above case, Gary's mother needed to listen to her son's feelings and concerns. There was a lot of anger over his father's death and she needed to react with tolerance and understanding to that first. His feeling of depression could indeed be understood if she listened to him with empathy. Then she would begin to make a real connection, and only then would it be appropriate to bring in to herself the hope that was required. She needed help, and healthcare professionals can feel helpless too in what appear to be intractable problems. By being hopeful in any situation we create opportunities for positive outcomes. Gary's depression did improve over months, and he began to get on better with his mother.

Enthusiasm

Enthusiasm is being optimistic
And is boundless energy and love of life.
Enthusiasm creates enthusiasm,
It encourages the faint-hearted, attracting friends.
Enthusiasm feels good, can achieve anything, and has no limits.

When we feel well, we are fully of energy. We wake in the morning excited about the day ahead, and see each new experience as being full of wonder. Perhaps we have all felt like this at some time, but the feeling is difficult to sustain. It requires perseverance; sticking at the task.

The starting point to generating more enthusiasm is to be optimistic. Search for the best, expect good outcomes, look on the bright side of life. Only by thinking these thoughts can it happen. Remember: actions follow thoughts.

We all know how the infectious enthusiasm of others can lift our spirits but to someone depressed, it can serve to underline feelings of inadequacy. We need to be sensitive to how they are by not talking enthusiastically but quietly embodying enthusiasm. Enthusiasm really works best at these subtle levels.

Humour

Laughter is the lubricant for joy
And loosens restrictions, dissolving embarrassment.
Humour heals wounds, and lightens loads,
It creates friendships.
Humour must be taken seriously.

Jack is an old priest who, when feeling down, goes out to a video shop and hires his favourite humorous videos. He sits at first, hardly raising a smile, but as the evening goes on starts to laugh heartily. By the end of the evening he can laugh at how seriously he takes himself. It may well seem to you that the last thing one would want to do when depressed is start laughing, but laughter is a medicine that works well.

I know an American doctor who takes fun very seriously. He is building a silly hospital; so silly, that he dresses up as a clown and does not charge patients. His hospital provides all the usual medical care, but also provides lots of entertainment, and encourages the patients to join in parties and play silly games.

We need to remember, even as adults wishing to pursue a spiritual path, that we must play and have fun. There should be a lightness on our journey; and the best way to do that is through humour and laughter. Fun is a serious matter.

Fourteen ways to overcome depression.

1   Accept you are depressed. Make time and take stock.

2   Accept change. Ask yourself why now; and where is the meaning in the depression.

3   Learn to trust that things will get better.

4   Think positively.

5   Make a recovery plan for each day, week, year.

6   Draw the depression.

7   Follow the light.

8   Find inner peace.

9   How would you like things to be?

10   Create your vision of a better world.

11   Focus on your inner positive qualities.

12   Trust that there is a compassionate, greater being.

13   Soak up beauty.

14   Bring the qualities of hope, enthusiasm and humour into your life.

Attachment

· ·

When the aim is optimum health, one of the main challenges is to learn to release the negative attribute of attachment. This does not mean selling up everything we own, but being less dependent on possessions.

Everyone has basic needs: water, food, clothing, shelter, love and affection. When need turns to a desire for more than we require to survive, that is when attachment develops. This desire can only bring temporary satisfaction.

It was five years since she had been burgled and Mrs Feist was still feeling low. She felt tired and irritable most of the time, was sleeping poorly, and had become obsessive about her security. The burglars had done a thorough job. The electrical equipment, her jewels and most of her furniture were taken during a break-in to her house. At first she was angry and indignant; then she became depressed. Although not a wealthy woman, she took great pride in her possessions, and replacing them using the insurance money did not help to lessen her depression.

The response following theft is similar to that following any loss. There are the negative feelings of anger, depression, guilt and worry, plus the sense of sorrow. It takes time to work through such loss, but five years is abnormal. In this case it was her attachment not only to her jewels that prevented her recovering: she wanted to hold on to her anger and her feelings of outrage. She was unwilling to let go of the anger and depression in the same way as she was unwilling to let go of her emotional attachment to her belongings.

Besides possessions we may also have attachments to other things such as alcohol, drugs, gambling and cigarettes. We are all familiar with the misuse of alcohol, drugs and smoking, as examples of substances that can lead to wanting more, with the expectation that they will satisfy that pleasure. Of course they do not, and in some people lead to a craving for more, even when it becomes obvious they seriously affect their health. Dependency and addiction are not easy problems to overcome.

Emotional attachment

Besides obvious dependencies such as alcohol, there is our emotional dependence on people. This is a difficult one as we all get nourishment from relationships. The problems occur in relationships of any kind when they are based on emotional needs rather than mutual support. The task is to loosen these emotional ties to allow us to become who we truly are. It is not easy to do this, especially after a lifetime habit. After all, the final act of letting go completely is to be ready to give up life itself without a sense of loss, and in doing so gain a sense of freedom.

John **was forty-two** when he was diagnosed as having liver cancer. He underwent chemotherapy and as a result became so ill that he had to give up his job. He had worked hard to reach a senior position with the water board, and had to resign from that. In addition he had to stop playing golf, curtail his social life, and relinquish voluntary positions he had held in charity organisations. He only had two years to live if he was lucky.

Later, during a consultation at the surgery, he told me that despite all his loss he would not have wished anything to be different. He was letting go of many of the things he had previously thought important, but had come to realise now they were not so important. He was preparing to let go of people as well; not that he loved them less, but was learning to become less emotionally dependent on them. He told me he was having to face that he had to give up life too. Through this experience he became more free, and each day became more intense. He said that if he had not had the cancer and had lived another thirty years, he would never have reached the same feeling of freedom he now had.

Attachment to others: jealousy

Jealousy can be at the root of many people's health problems. There is a wariness in their look, a secretiveness in what is said, and a reluctance to divulge the problem. Jealousy is essentially attachment to such a degree that we feel we need the other person so much, we become suspicious of anyone who may be attracting their attention, and so competing for our affection. It is the fear of the loss of that affection that becomes the obsession. Jealousy can become quite an extreme type of attachment to a person and, like all negative qualities, increases in power if it is suppressed.

Janet looked tense as she walked into the surgery. She surprised me, as I remembered the last time she had attended with her husband they had seemed such a happy couple. She said she had lost weight, was miserable, and felt sick after meals. It had all begun around six months ago, when her husband had begun to work late at the office. She paused and with some reluctance she went on to say that she secretly suspected that he was having an affair with his new secretary, but dared not mention anything as she had no proof. She was jealous of this woman and imagined ways in which she could catch them together. It had reached the point that when he came home from work she accused him of all sorts of things without directly referring to her suspicions. Now she was aware that their marriage was at risk. Sharing her secret fears enabled her to realise it was her own jealousy that was making her ill.

Letting go of jealousy can take courage; it is an act of surrendering one's pride. We make all sorts of excuses to avoid bringing things into the open like: It would look silly. Everyone will laugh at me. I will be rejected. It is too late.

It is a risk to change, but it is one gamble worth taking, because there will be just one winner: and that will be you.

Attachment to self: pride

It is natural for each one of us to want to improve ourselves: to improve our skills, our knowledge, to become better individuals. It is right to be proud of our achievements, but inflated self-esteem leads to pride. When it is a belief that our view is correct and others are inferior, that is arrogance. Pride gets in the way of recovery from illness in many instances. It can stop us from beginning to accept that we are ill in the first place.

Another kind of pride is spiritual pride, in which people who profess a special spiritual knowledge seek to teach others. Think of those religious groups who come to your door peddling the writings of their leader with an evangelical zeal as though they were the only truth, and their mission was to convert you to their way of thinking.

Sarah Parkins came to tell me that she had been to a charismatic healing service, and as a result had been able to stop her arthritic drugs. She was full of enthusiasm, and recounted how the preacher had touched her on the forehead, causing her to fall to the ground. When she came round, the pain and stiffness in her hands were gone, and everyone around proclaimed it was a miracle as she could walk without her sticks. Several days later I saw her and she had her sticks once again, but she said the pain was definitely better. Three weeks later she started her medication again as her pain had returned.

It is understandable that people should seek cures; but it is best to beware of the charismatic preacher and the cults that offer 'easy' solutions. I sometimes see vulnerable people lured by easy answers only to suffer disillusionment later. The spiritual truth is found along a personal, sometimes lonely, journey but that is where true healing occurs. However, do look for people to help and guide you; they will surely appear.

Attachment to illness: the sick role

When we are ill we evoke sympathy in others; and having people caring for us is of great benefit to our recovery. However some people find the role of being sick so comforting that they lose the motivation to get better. They adopt the attitude of a victim: 'Poor me, I am hopeless, and helpless, and cannot manage without your help.' In short, they become attached to their illness. Unfortunately they attract an equally dependent group of people who need to be needed. They then fit into the role of rescuer. This victim and rescuer role is one for all doctors and health workers to beware of. The third person who goes to make the triangle is the persecutor and is the one the victim blames, real or imagined, for all his ills. This triangle of three types of people involved in sickness leads nowhere unless the dependence they have on each other is recognised. The purpose of an illness is to give an indication that something is out of balance. It is not a matter of adapting to the imbalance, but of listening to the message in the symptoms of the illness, and changing.

Mrs Quinn was a blind widow living on her own. When she heard about the healer working at our surgery she decided to come as she thought it could help her eyesight. She attended on a weekly basis, and slowly her vision began to improve. Then one day her neighbour said that if she continued to do so well she would soon not be needing her blind person's pension any more. Her vision deteriorated soon after that conversation, and she stopped attending the healing sessions.

The meaning of attachment

Thirst, hunger, warmth, sex, are very strong physical drives in all humans, and the first three are essential for personal survival, and sex for the survival of the species. So they undoubtedly have a clear function. Care and companionship are necessary for our emotional needs. For our spiritual needs we only need love.

It is when we shift from need to desire that these attachments increasingly prevent us from finding optimum healing. The change in attitude that requires to be made is from ownership to stewardship. This is when we find the true meaning.

Think of the things we own not as ours, but as things we have been given to look after. We are only temporary carers and as such we have a duty to look after the items we care for while they are in our possession, before the next person uses them. They will still be present long after we are dead. Stewardship is the spiritual approach of caring for possessions.

Recently a neighbour of mine wanted to plant some fast-growing trees on the border of our garden. I felt this would spoil my garden; it would reduce the light and put flowering shrubs in the shade. I could see us entering a dispute over our rights as landowners, and employing lawyers at great expense. This ill feeling on my part continued for some weeks, until I began to reflect on how such a small thing could annoy me so much when compared to the general scheme of things. We would both be dead in twenty or thirty years, and the house and garden would still be there. Indeed the land had been there for many thousands of years, and would still be for many more. When I took the longer term view my attitude began to change from being defensive and confrontational to being more co-operative. So I wrote to her suggesting we planted a slower growing beech hedge, which would enhance the look of both gardens over a longer term. The change of attitude on my part was critical in settling the dispute in a friendly manner.

The following exercises are all ways of letting go, and loosening the ties that bind you to things and people. The purpose is not to leave you feeling stripped bare, but to create a nakedness that reveals the true you; a beautiful being, free of any attachments.

Letting go of possessions

Imagine you are at home, comfortably sitting in your favourite chair. The door bell rings and you open the door. Standing there are people in uniforms, saying that you have to leave your home immediately. It is an emergency. An earthquake is expected soon, and the whole area is being evacuated. You only have a few minutes to put some belongings into a small case. What would you take?

You are taken to safety in a ship, and eventually you are set ashore on a small deserted island. What use are the things you have taken?

This exercise helps us judge the true value to us of some of our material possessions, and how we could manage without them.

Make a list of what you consider to be your most important and essential possessions. Next to this list, write down why they are essential. Now ask yourself if these things are really so inherently pleasing to you that you would suffer if you no longer had them. We do tend to exaggerate the importance of some things. You may be able, on reflection, to score a few of them off that now seem not so essential.

From time to time, in a very practical way, we all throw out clothes, books and some household goods. We give them away to jumble sales, to charities or put them in the bin. I often feel a sense of relief after such an exercise; and perhaps a certain lightness. It is even more rewarding if someone else has benefited because I have given them away. Do not be a hoarder; have regular clear-outs, and in that way you will become less dependent on your goods.

Letting go of people

Do not think I am going to recommend you dump all your friends! In a similar way list your friends. It could be an idea to include your partner, parents and children on your list. Alongside the list write why you need them. Be as honest as you can. Some of the reasons may be because you value their opinion, or they make you feel secure, or they make you laugh. Of course that is not the only reason you are friends or have strong connections. But if you do have strong needs of them how would you feel if they left the area, or you were not likely to see them for a long time?

Such emotional needs can lead to jealousy and suspicion, and may well be getting in the way of your present relationship. I am not advocating that you become distant and indifferent to them, but that your relationships should be grounded on mutual respect of their true values, and not of your expectations. The bonds we form with others should be bonds of love, the love given without conditions, without desire. Not the love of wanting, but the unselfish love of giving. This is the love that does not grieve with loss, but gives thanks for what has been.

Letting go of pride

This time, list all your own attributes: your physical and mental skills, all the various things that contribute to make your personality. Are you good at sport or at arranging flowers, do you play a musical instrument, have dexterity skills, have a good voice, cook, repair a bicycle? List all the attributes that you feel make you who you are. Now think how you would manage without any one of them, or indeed without all of them.

Letting go of life

Imagine you know you only have a few hours to live. What good are your possessions now: your wealth, your car and house? What good is your position in society, or the awards you have collected? Who do you need, and why? These questions will help you understand what attachments you have, not only to material goods but to people, and perhaps to your own self-importance. At death you cannot take any of these with you.

Peacefulness

Accumulating possessions does not lead to happiness. It leads to wanting more. Neither does dependence on things or people. Optimum healing is to do with being free of attachment, and is based on our state of mind, not on what we own, how we see ourselves, or who we know. We need to learn to loosen our attachments, and as they are shed, our own inner peace will begin to shine through. This letting go is like peeling off layers of an onion to reveal our true inner core of peacefulness.

Finding Peace

TAKE A WALK
Go for a walk in a park. If you are lucky, walk by the seashore, in a forest, or anywhere close to nature. Observe closely everything you see. The way the light plays on the leaves or waves, the sounds, the different shades of colour, shape of trees, patterns in the sand.

There is so much beauty to observe and enjoy in abundance in nature, yet we do not have to desire or own it all to be happy. Appreciating the beauty of nature is a route towards inner peace. It brings the realisation that there is enough to go round for everyone without needing to own what we enjoy.

DETACHMENT

Find a quiet spot in which you will not be interrupted and sit comfortably, gently relaxing in the way described in the chapter on worry. Once your body is relaxed, your breathing easy, let your mind go quiet. Using your imagination see yourself as a small point of light, situated just behind your eyes, in the middle of your forehead. Slowly and easily, that point moves upwards, above where you are sitting, into the vast silence of space. You are looking down on to the earth below. You leave behind concerns about your possessions and the needs you have of others. You are detached and experience a deep peace. Stay as long as you like experiencing how it feels to be free of all desires, needs and possessions. This is peace, freedom and happiness.

Spiritual awareness and possessiveness

Soul consciousness

To free ourselves from the desires of the 'I' we must begin to listen to who we truly are, and tune in to our soul nature. It is not a matter of ignoring all the senses and desires that are part of being human, but of acknowledging them for what they are; not letting them overwhelm us and take control. If we stand aside and view them from a soul perspective we see that they only bring temporary satisfaction.

At forty-three years old, Bob Beauly was unlikely to work again. He had chronic backache as a result of an injury at work. Not only did he have a serious problem with his back, he had made up his mind that he was not going to get better. It suited him not to have the responsibility of work and he fell easily into the sick role. He was the sort of man who prided himself in getting his own way. He said he wanted the pain to go from his back, and seemed frustrated that the numerous doctors he had seen were not able to cure his pain. The trouble was that he saw himself solely in terms of his bodily needs. If he was hungry, he had some food; if cold, he kept warm. If he wanted a car, he worked hard to buy it; if in pain, he took something to relieve it. This view of being just a body with needs and desires limited Bob's ability to tackle his back pain.

Bob identified only with his ego. The ego is the 'I' which is where our thoughts are focused when we are concerned with our needs and desires. It leads to a limited and self-centred existence. Like Bob, most of us have probably spent most of our life operating from this position of ego consciousness. When we shift the focus of our thinking to a soul within a body things can begin to look different. It is then opportunities open for real change.

Bob's backache did not improve. He was very unhappy, and he became more and more annoyed with the medical profession's inability to help him. His frustration led him to seek the help of a massage therapist, and very slowly he began to make the connection between mind and body. Over months she gradually introduced the idea of positive thinking, and he became open to the spiritual dimension of his being. He began to explore some of the alternative approaches to his problem by reading and attending classes. Four years after the injury he was working again part time in a different job; and more importantly he was much more content with himself and the world.

God consciousness

With this looking inward to our own soul consciousness, it seems that as our awareness deepens we also begin to look outward. There is an expansion in our awareness and there is a sense of connection to the soul of the universe.

This awareness, which I have called God consciousness, is achieved through communication in three ways: prayer, meditation and contemplation on the qualities of God. Just to open up a conversation with this universal being as a friend, a guide, and a trusted companion is to enter into *prayer*. Sharing His presence in stillness is meditation. Observing the beauty of nature and His being is contemplation.

'**G**od is by** my shoulder,' was what Margaret Langholm told me through short gasping breaths as she faced her last journey towards death. She said that she thought of Him as a travelling companion who showed her kindness, patience and compassion.

At Margaret's funeral those were the qualities on most people's lips when they spoke of her. I remember her dying with a smile on her face despite the physical suffering she must have experienced. Margaret took no pride in her possessions, or in her social position. At the end she had no attachment to her physical body, and was also able to let that go with ease. She had achieved much in her life with her work and her family, and showed a quiet humility. It seemed that the qualities she saw in God became part of her. She lived the greater part of her life, particularly towards the end, in that God consciousness.

Collective consciousness

One can view soul consciousness as looking inward, God consciousness as looking out and upward, and collective consciousness as looking around. It is seeing that we are connected to every other human being, to every other thing, living and material in the world.

If that is a view we can accept, and can get a sense of, one can begin to realise: 'By changing ourselves we begin to change the world.' It is also true that trying to change the world into a better place will help to change us.

John was what** you would have called 'a grumpy old man'. Nothing pleased him. His tablets upset him, he objected if he had to wait, and he complained that no one cared for him. Shortly after they moved to a flat on the seafront five years ago his wife had died and he felt that was the hospital's fault. A neighbour who knew John was aware that he had been a keen gardener, and approached him to suggest he help out with a conservation group doing some tree planting. Soon John was joining them most weekends, and later told me it was the best thing he ever did. Certainly, he lost his negative attitude. It was not only the companionship and getting out into the country that he enjoyed, but also the feeling that he was contributing to future generations through the work he was doing. He would often say to those watching him work: 'It will be your children's children who will benefit from my labours!'

This is the concept of stewardship practically applied to a local environmental situation. We come to the land on birth, and will leave it behind on death. The attitude of stewardship is to care for, and to try to improve the environment during our lifetime. It is our task to leave this world in a better state than we found it. This is the spiritual attitude: to ask not 'What can I get?' but 'How can I be of service?' We only have to look at how planning in towns and the countryside is often for short-term gain, with little thought for future generations.

The North American Indians ask of themselves and others, 'How can we humans own the stones, the water, the earth?' They argue that they have been present for many millions of years, and will be around for many millions more when we are dead. Our short lifespan pales into insignificance in comparison. Even the life of a country, be it a hundred or a thousand years, is nothing compared to the life of the land. So when building a house or road, plan not only for the next generation, but imagine how it will look in seven generations hence.

IMAGINE THE EARTH

Imagine you are in a spaceship circling the earth. You look down on this amazing and beautiful sight. The vast blue seas, the land of browns and greens, the streaks of white cloud over the surface. You can recognise the shapes of continents, and try to fit in the countries to these huge land masses. Then you realise you can see no borders between them. The planet earth is one great whole. That is the reality of how it has always been. Up in space you are detached, but at the same time care deeply about the earth, and every living being. Now think of the people on the earth below with love and understanding. And send that energy of love back to the earth that has given so much to you.

Spiritual qualities for attachment

What are the positive qualities you would choose to overcome the negative energy of attachment? I have chosen generosity, humility and discipline.

Generosity

> Generosity lightens the spirit
> And creates goodwill.
> Generosity breaks barriers,
> It is an opportunity to loosen attachments.
> Generosity is the road to freedom.

It is said that if you give with ill-will, the ill-will returns to you, but if you give with joy, the joy returns. When we give money to charity, or a compliment to a friend, it is not how much we give or what we say that matters, it is the intention that is important. Sharing what you have with joy will bring happiness to both the giver and the receiver.

Perhaps what is less well appreciated is that many of us as receiver must learn to receive gifts graciously, neither burdening the giver with profuse praise nor ignoring them completely. With such an attitude between giver and receiver the gift can be seen as a sharing of the natural abundance of the earth.

Beware of seeking praise; that is a different type of attachment, wanting people to respect you for what you do, and not what you are.

ACTING GENEROUSLY

Performing spontaneous acts of generosity is a very practical way to overcome the meanness of being possessive. Make a donation to a charity. Give away something you really value; then observe how you feel. Perhaps at first you will have a sense of loss and emptiness, but remember this emptiness can also be a feeling of lightness; an offloading of a burden, a release that leads to freedom.

Besides being generous with our money or our material goods, we can be generous in other ways. We give of ourselves by being generous with our time, giving compliments to others. It allows us to be more expansive and open.

We cannot truly learn generosity until we learn to be generous with ourselves, mainly by being kinder and more forgiving to ourselves.

Humility

Humility is the acceptance of others
And eliminates all attachments.
Humility is at the depth of self-esteem.
It makes you smile.
Humility leads to service.

Achieving humility is difficult. There is a fine line first between confidence and arrogance and second between assertiveness and bullying. It takes considerable effort to find this balance, to be vigilant against jealousy and pride. I fail every day, then I remember to be generous with myself. Forgive my uselessness and try better next time.

At a private insurance medical Mr Jackson was found to be diabetic. I advised him to lose weight and change his lifestyle. He was a proud man and very successful in his work. He was reluctant to alter his lifetime habits of rich food and wine, and as a result his diabetes was poorly controlled. Some years later he became blind. His pride had blocked the good advice he was given. A touch of humility may well have made him more open to change.

We sometimes have to learn humility the hard way. Often we arrive at humility through ignorance. How many times have we criticised someone, only to feel ashamed when we have learned what they have suffered?

To get in touch with all our core values is a theme which I

encourage throughout this book. Practising these in our daily life allows us to experience the power of humility.

You may know of some people who have inspired ideas, and begin to believe that the ideas are their own. This is spiritual pride. Inspired thoughts do not come *from* us but *through* us. We are simply vehicles, so it is no good thinking ourselves to be geniuses just because we have channelled a good idea.

Glamour and fame are also sought by some spiritual leaders; a sure sign that we should examine their teachings carefully. Humility is the quality which frees us from believing that we are better than others; it is the quality seen in true spiritual leaders, wanting to help others without seeking fame or praise.

Discipline

Discipline is being honest.
It is needed to implement our vision.
Discipline requires willpower.
It tests our resolve, and requires perseverance.
Discipline is the key to develop all other spiritual qualities.

When I have asked people to score on a list of spiritual qualities as I did in the introduction the quality which most people scored lowest in was discipline. We may think, even know in our hearts, that it is right for us to be kind, generous and compassionate; but to have the discipline to bring these positive qualities into action is another matter.

Most people who smoke know it is not good for their health, and many make plans to stop. I used to smoke and planned to stop many times. From the first time I tried to stop it took me two years to succeed. Lack of self-discipline usually let me down, despite knowledge of all the risks to my health. The same is true with other health measure such as losing weight, taking more exercise or cutting down on alcoholic drinks. We start off with good intentions, but we soon begin to waver in our resolve.

It is not only in measures to improve physical health that one needs discipline. Despite my deep conviction of the value of regular meditation, I still find it difficult to practise regularly. Self-discipline is the most difficult quality to integrate, and is the one quality at which we need to work hardest. If you fail, do not fall into the trap of thinking it cannot be done, or it is not for you. Analyse why you were not successful, set yourself a new goal and try again. Do not be harsh on yourself; after all, if your intentions are pure you will be successful. Most people struggle with self-discipline.

A spiritual guide to successful personal relationships

1   When I look at you, I see a peaceful being.

2   When we are close there remains some space between us.

3   I am tolerant of your shortcomings.

4   I see you in me; and me in you.

5   I allow you time alone to find your way without me.

6   When you are not here, I think of your positive qualities and try to bring these into myself.

7   People I dislike are sent to teach me.

8   I will not criticise you until I have walked a hundred miles in your shoes.

9   I forgive you, just as a loving mother would.

10   When I know you are not coming back I will cut the cord that binds us, and let you go free.

Worry

The mind can sometimes seem in a turmoil of worry; thought after thought keeps crowding in until there seems no more room to contain them all. Such concerns seem overpowering to the extent that they continually interfere with our thinking, despite us telling ourselves that we are worrying unnecessarily.

What starts as a simple concern can soon turn into a major worry. To be concerned about ourselves and others is normal. Concern about illness, finance, work and about our loved ones is natural; but concern with fear equals worry. We worry about those close to us when they are not with us: 'Are they safe?' 'Have they been killed in a car crash?' and so on. We worry about ourselves. 'Have I got a serious illness?' 'Am I a good enough person?' 'Do people like me?' We worry about money, status, our job. In fact, we worry about everything.

Mr Tell was a chronic worrier who inhaled some smoke and thought he had a stomach ulcer. When his wife had headaches, he thought she might develop a stroke. When he had abdominal pains, it was appendicitis. A cough was tuberculosis, a nail infection gangrene. He worried about becoming ill; and all these thoughts of illness and the possible outcomes tormented his mind. His attendance at the surgery nearly always followed a friend's illness. On each visit, he had to have an examination and full explanation before he was reassured.

Persistent worry is well known to cause many illnesses; a duodenal ulcer is a classic example. The worry starts in the mind, and is transmitted through the nervous system linking the brain and the stomach. The stomach produces more acid, which over a long period leads to ulceration of the duodenum in the lower part of the stomach. Not only is this very uncomfortable for the sufferer, but it can also be life-threatening if the ulcer perforates the stomach wall. Other problems caused by worry include tension headaches, irritable bowel, palpitations, insomnia, jumpy legs and many more. Such illnesses are known as psychosomatic: *psycho* = mind; *soma* = body.

Sylvia was a lady who took on everyone's problems as well as her own. She complained of flushing and sweating and after listing her current worries for twenty minutes, she said at the door as she was leaving, 'I get overheated about things a lot of the time.'

At that moment the penny dropped for her. She realised that it was the state of her mind that was causing her symptoms.

Stress and anxiety

Stress leads to worry; and what is stressful in one person is not in another. It is very much to do with our mental attitude towards problems. If we see changes as problems, we will have problems, and experience worry. If we see changes in life as challenges to be faced and solved, we will grow through the experience, and not suffer worry.

Some of the biggest stress factors that most people go through during their life include: a family bereavement, divorce, moving house, and leaving home. Happy events such as marriage, the birth of a child, and even Christmas can also cause considerable stress. Other changes that figure high on the list of stress factors are: loss of a job, promotion at work, illness and retirement. Patients will consult their general practitioner often with seemingly quite trivial reasons when the underlying cause is stress.

Jackie was a very able twenty-seven-year-old store manager, who over recent months could not understand why she could not relax when she came home at night. She had busy days, but enjoyed her work. Financially she felt secure, and everything was going well with her long-term boyfriend with whom she shared the house. I went through all the usual stress factors, but together we could not come up with an answer. I changed the approach and asked her to make a list of all the things she felt were achievable this year, and what she could do to make her life happier. She surprised me by reacting enthusiastically to this idea, and went off to try it out. I never found out what it was that had inspired her, but the next occasion that she consulted me she reported that, as a result of making the list and thinking through her priorities, she felt much better. She had shifted her view and at some level could understand her problem.

Everyone has the capacity to heal themselves, and as a doctor my job is to help patients find their own way, not tell them what to do.

Anxiety is how we experience worry, and is something with which we are all familiar. The sudden rush of adrenaline in the bloodstream when faced with a threat causes symptoms of anxiety. The heart suddenly begins to pump fast, the mouth becomes dry, the palms of our hands sweat, our muscles tense ready for action. Even our facial expression changes, and the pupils of our eyes dilate. This is known as the 'fight or flight mechanism' and was vital to man for his survival in primitive times. It is still useful now for emergency situations which require an immediate response, such as jumping out of the path of an oncoming bus. People who do worry a lot will often complain of some of these 'fight or flight' symptoms, not just as something temporary, but as being chronic. Neck tension, band-like headache, palpitations of the heart and dryness in the mouth are common complaints in patients with anxiety.

Marie was a full-time lecturer at a local college as well as being a mother of two children. Her complaint was a muscle pain in her shoulder that she'd had for some months; she said she wanted something to rub into it. She did not look her usual enthusiastic self, and she asked at the door on her way out if she could have something to soothe her tension. I invited her back to talk some more, and she talked of the band-like headaches she experienced while working. She had become more irritable in recent months and her husband had noticed she was grinding her teeth in her sleep.

She admitted she had many worries including mortgage payments, shortage of money, and staff sickness at work. She said there were no problems in her relationship with her husband and children. However I had seen her young daughter with several episodes of severe abdominal pains that had been investigated and no cause found. She describe her main problem as the inability to stop her mind racing. She could not stop worrying, and was keen to have some help.

She saw one of the healers at our surgery who helped her experience a deep sense of relaxation that began to help her to feel better. This recovery was not simply getting rid of the symptoms of tiredness, but was the kick-start to her spiritual journey. She felt better with herself, although her problems were far from over. Incidentally, after Marie started practising relaxation her daughter's abdominal pains went. Worry in one member of a family can be transmitted to another, causing them also to suffer symptoms.

Hyperventilation is a common symptom of anxiety where the breathing is rapid and shallow. It results in blowing off too much carbon dioxide and chemical changes in the blood cause muscle spasms.

This happened to a forty-eight-year-old financial advisor who woke up during the night with chest pains. He was breathing very fast, and was alarmed by the 'pins and needles' in his face and hands. He had suffered panic attacks before, but the chest ache really worried him, as he knew that his father died of a heart attack when fifty-three. He went to see a Harley Street heart specialist and underwent extensive medical investigations, including an arteriogram to outline his heart blood vessels. All the tests were declared normal, but he still had the symptoms. It was then that he accepted that he had been hyperventilating and it must be due to worry – and that he had to do something about it, even if that did mean changing his whole lifestyle. Which he did by going part time at work, and took up painting. A good start!

Dealing with worry

If you are a worrier, do not despair. The habit of worrying is a pattern of thinking, and understanding that gives hope that it is something you can change. The optimum healing approach is to look for meaning, and develop spiritual qualities; to see the goals as not just eliminating worry but increasing spiritual awareness and finding inner peace.

The meaning of worry

Just as anger has the purpose of raising our energy, worry serves the purpose of alerting us to danger. It brings the body into a state of readiness, the mind alert and the body tensed ready for action. However, if the action does not follow and we continue in this state of arousal, the effect will be harmful and result in illness.

In many ways, perhaps the purpose of worry is to make us feel uncomfortable. It alerts us to our own state of imbalance by producing symptoms. Rather than try to ignore or fight against these signs, we should accept and welcome them, for they indicate that something is out of balance and needs changing.

Another meaning may be to draw to our attention the illness itself. Patients tend to describe their illness in the very words that perfectly describe their underlying feelings. Where the discomfort is sited in the body will give a clue. The body speaks to us of feelings. We have to learn to interpret what it is saying literally and at the same time symbolically. However there is no fixed list of symptoms which identify one underlying problem. The best approach is to ask oneself if a particular symptom is literally pointing to the real problem. Symptoms give us a clue to discover the cause of our illness, and to restore our personal balance. At our deep spiritual level there is drive and desire to reach harmony and wholeness.

Ways to overcome worry

See concerns as challenges

Worry is concern coupled with fear. Thus if we are able to change our approach so that we can be concerned without fear, there will be no worry. It is our attitude that determines whether or not we suffer from worry. When we begin to think positively fear is removed so that concerns then become challenges.

However, viewing concerns as challenges does not come easily to most people. Even when we recognise the need to change our attitude, actually doing so can often prove too difficult. It is relatively easy to change external things, but to change within ourselves is infinitely more difficult. Think of it in this way: worry is not something we are born with and have to live with for the rest of our lives; it is not part of our essential nature. It may have attached itself to our personality through continual habit. Nevertheless such habits of thought can be shed with practice. Understanding this concept is only the first step; putting it into practice is a path which will likely require many steps.

Spiritual post

A **mother of two** young children told me how she overcomes the constant worry she has about them when they are not with her. Previously every time she thought about them she used to worry irrationally. Now when such thoughts arise she tries to see them clearly in her mind's eye at whatever they may be doing. She then imagines a beautiful golden light in the scene she has created, and surrounds them with a ball of this light. The light that she sends is her love for her children. She calls this 'spiritual post'.

This method is a very practical way of dealing with worrying thoughts. When such a thought arises in your mind, rather than trying to get rid of it, hold on to it. If it is a concern about a person hold an image of that person in your mind's eye. Try to capture the essence of that person. At the same time, imagine a golden sphere of light and see that light as representing love; a warm, generous, unconditional love. Now send that love to the person you are worrying about, and surround them with it. Try to practise this simple idea yourself over the next few days towards any worry that comes to mind. Not only will you be sending protection to that person; it will also make you feel better.

This way of dealing with worrying thoughts can be applied to anybody or anything. For example, if you are frightened of flying surround the whole plane in a golden or white light within your mind's eye. In doing so you are creating protection at a deep level.

Abdominal breathing

Breathing into a paper bag is one of the well-known ways of overcoming hyperventilation. For a more permanent result, a very simple exercise is to use abdominal breathing. Many people, particularly those who suffer with hyperventilation problems, breathe mainly from the upper chest. You can check this yourself by taking a deep breath and observing which part of your chest inflates. The diaphragm is the main breathing muscle, which you can feel easily if you lie on your back and watch your stomach go up and down. Place your hands on the upper part of your abdomen and feel them move; they will be gently lifted up and down. What you are actually feeling under your hands is the diaphragm moving with each breath. Take a few deep breaths at first to establish the rhythm, then allow it to fall to its natural rate up and down. Breathe through your nose and count your breaths. Normally at rest we take between twelve and sixteen breaths per minute. Watch the breathing rather than try to control it; this is the most natural thing in the world, but at first it can seem quite difficult. It is a good ideal to practise for five minutes before going to sleep at night. It is a wonderful way of relaxing for everyone, and it is particularly helpful for those who do hyperventilate.

Peacefulness

To discover a truly peaceful state is the goal of every individual wishing to achieve optimum health; and is all the more urgent for anyone who suffers from worry, as they are in an opposite state from peacefulness.

All the symptoms of worry – tremor, a racing pulse, a churning stomach and tense neck muscles – have their origin in an agitated mind. Thoughts move fast, coming and going; then running around in circles, finally ending up all jumbled. New thoughts continue to arise, adding to the inner turmoil, and there seems to be no relief. Even when asleep, the mind remains in a state of constant activity. Under these circumstances it seems to control us and worry takes over. But our mind is the one thing over which we can have control.

It works both ways: a deep unease at our spiritual level affects our thinking, and an uneasy mind affects the deeper spiritual levels. If we really do want to get to grips with our problem seriously and permanently, we need to set time aside each day to give the matter proper attention.

Most people will have some idea as to the sort of thing that they personally find relaxing. Walking the dog, listening to music or soaking in a hot bath are all examples. Exercises involving tensing and relaxing muscles are a useful start to relaxation and are described in many self-help books. Some of the popular Eastern approaches such as Yoga, Tai Chi, and Qui Quong are all very helpful in providing relaxation. But ultimately it depends on the state of your mind as to whether or not you are able to achieve that deep state of peace.

Finding Peace

SITTING QUIETLY: RELAXING THE BODY

The first issue is when and where to practise. Try to choose a place in the house where you have a chance of being quiet: a spare bedroom, the corner of a lounge, or any area in which you can sit undisturbed. The best time of day is early morning, when not only the house but also the whole neighbourhood is quiet. However, evening is fine; or for that matter, any time will do. I generally like the hour between 5 and 6 p.m. because the rest of the family is watching *Neighbours* on the television! If you do have difficulty in sitting still, start off with setting aside ten minutes at a time, and increase this further by stages up to thirty minutes. After some practice you will find that you can sit up to an hour at a stretch.

Having decided on the 'where' and 'when', the next step is the 'how'. It does not really matter too much how you sit, as long as you are comfortable. If you use a seat it is best if you have your feet uncrossed and flat on the floor. If you prefer to sit on the floor with your legs crossed, a cushion under your bottom helps to keep a straight spine. I find it useful to imagine that a string is pulling gently up from the centre of the skull, rather like a puppet string; this not only straightens the spine, but also relaxes the shoulders. Your hands should rest relaxed on your lap. Close your eyes, but keep them open just enough to let in some light so you do not become too sleepy. Just sitting in this posture is enough to help you begin to feel relaxed.

Soft background music playing may help to create a calm environment. It should also stop you being distracted by other noises. Creating your own routine builds up the atmosphere to make each session increasingly more powerful.

STILLING THE MIND: WATCHING THE BREATH

Control of the breath is the key to good relaxation; it makes a connection between mind and body. Breathe through your nose and allow the breath to be easy, finding its own rhythm. Simply focus your attention on the air causing a slight draught through your nostrils. Imagine your breathing is like the waves on a seashore. As it goes out, so go all your worries. As it draws in, it brings calm. In order to stop your mind wandering, count the breaths, from one to five then back down to zero to start with. If you can count up to eight and back without losing your place, you are doing very well. Remember, this is not a competition; do not be hard on yourself. If you make a mistake, don't worry, just start again.

STILLING THE MIND: USING THE MIND

Sitting comfortably in a quiet place, breathing regularly with the body relaxed, your mind will be experiencing a sense of calm. You may be so calm that you are beginning to fall off to sleep. However, while this may be a useful way to help to relax yourself before going off to sleep at night, for this purpose try to keep your thoughts clear. Continue by emptying your mind of all external distractions like a door banging, or bodily distractions like an itch or ache. Then give up trying. Perhaps a calm image will help, like seeing the calm of a surface of a lake. A forest lit up by moonlight. A deserted beach. The absolute quietness of outer space. Listen to the stillness, and then experience the peacefulness. This stillness should not be so much a dream-like state, but one of clarity, and being fully alive. This is the emptiness which is full, to which so many mystical writings refer. An emptiness that is full of peace.

STILLING THE MIND: CONNECTING WITH SPIRIT

People will differ in their own definitions and descriptions of what is true meditation. It has been described as 'like coming home', 'a peacefulness beyond silence', or 'meeting God'. Whatever is experienced as stillness at a spiritual level is clearly very personal, something beyond concepts and words.

As we continue the exercise of stilling the mind, one may begin to sense the part of you that is experiencing peacefulness. This is not just your body and mind, but a point that is the core of your nature. See this point as a small bright light. Once you have gained a sense of this point of light, see it separate from your body and move off into the vast emptiness of silence. You, as the point of light, approach another much stronger light. You realise that this light is the source of all peace; and it seems to resonate with you, making your peacefulness even more powerful. The supreme light welcomes and nourishes you; it is the embrace of finally returning home. This experience is meditation. Savour, inhale, breathe the experience.

When you feel ready, slowly see that point of light move gradually back within your body where you are sitting. Move your limbs gently so that you feel your hands on your lap and your feet on the ground. Open your eyes slowly and stretch your limbs. Take in everything in the room; and after a few minutes, when you feel ready, get up and return to your day, bringing into it the peacefulness you have just experienced.

Meditation is essentially simple but requires practice. If you intend to take it further there are many courses, books and tapes you will find useful.

At our surgery every year we hold an exam stress class for fifteen-year-olds who need help with relaxation. We offer them various techniques, but when we question them as to which one they found the most helpful, it is surprising to learn how often they answer that it is meditation.

FURTHER WAYS TO FIND PEACE IN A BUSY DAY

Telephone When a telephone rings on your desk, possibly interrupting something important you are doing, do not answer it immediately. Stop and take three deep, slow breaths before picking up the receiver. This will mean you will have calmed yourself before dealing with the interruption, and so can afford it your full attention without feeling annoyed.

Washing When you wash your hands, imagine that the water is washing away any negative attributes that you may have picked up. Having a shower using such imagery can also be truly refreshing. Another way to rid yourself of negativity is simply to shake it from your hands, or to brush it off your limbs.

Waiting If you have to wait for an appointment sit like stone, with limitless patience. Take advantage of the situation to calm yourself and become detached from your surroundings. Then, if there is a delay, you will be quite grateful for this interval in your day.

Traffic lights This is one of my favourites, because I used to get annoyed when the traffic lights had just turned to red as I approached in my car. Then someone told me that they were always grateful when that happened to them, as they knew they had at least one more minute undisturbed, and perhaps longer. Such moments can be a chance to remember who we truly are, and to turn inwards to our soul nature.

Cleaning teeth I like to think that when I am cleaning my teeth I am cleaning out all nasty words that were said that day. Once something unpleasant is said it cannot be unsaid. Bad words create a bad atmosphere, causing negativity.

Standing Again, if you have to stand and wait, for instance at a station for a train, feel both your feet firmly on the ground. Think of yourself as a tree that has strong deep roots into the ground. This really does give one a sense of being firmly rooted in life.

Walking Often in the office, most of the day is spent sitting. It is important from a physical and mental point of view to get up and move at least every half-hour, otherwise you will become very sluggish. From the spiritual aspect, when you do walk up a corridor or stair, do so slowly. Concentrate on your feet and the purposeful movement of your legs. This is how monks walked around their cloisters. The practice moves you out of your daily worries into a more peaceful sort of existence.

Toilet We British can be quite obsessive about the regularity of our bowel movements! So why not see this not simply as a necessary physical function, but also as a way of expelling emotional and spiritual rubbish along with our physical waste. Worry is a negative attribute so no useful purpose is served by holding on to it.

Travelling Sitting on a train is an ideal opportunity to take time for yourself. If it is a long journey, any or all of the exercises in this book can be practised. On a short journey, such as on the tube, try the exercise in which you fill yourself with light. Think of a golden beam of light entering your head and filling your whole body; then expanding to bring light to everyone in the carriage.

Spiritual awareness

Soul consciousness

We are mind, body, emotion and spirit. Worry is a constant distraction that invariably keeps us from paying attention to the spiritual part of who we truly are. It seems that our lives are full of busyness; from the moment we get up until we go to bed at night, we are constantly doing things, or thinking about doing things. But we are not human *doings*; we are human *beings*. We need to learn more how to be, and stop doing; we must make time to remember who we are inside. This busy-ness is not only at the physical level, but in our minds; even when we are in a physically quiet environment, our thoughts race round and round as though stuck in a groove: What plans do I have tomorrow? What have I forgotten to do? What did I do wrong yesterday? Such thoughts bring up new and old emotions with their associated anxieties and soon we will begin to feel the uneasiness in our body.

WHO AM I?

First, put some time aside to get acquainted with this person you live with all your life. Ten to fifteen minutes to start with each day will be enough. If possible find a quiet place. This can all be part of that same special time you schedule into the day, just for yourself. If you do begin to find this time is useful, treat yourself and allow more.

Next, you need to remove the labels that have been attached to yourself, such as your position in the family. A man typically takes the role of father, husband, son, provider; and a woman, mother, daughter, sister, home keeper. Similarly, the colour of your skin, your nationality, your political party or your job may be a role with which you identify, but they are not the essential you. Peel back the coverings that you have enfolded around yourself, or that have been imposed upon you. Underneath is a very unique and special individual.

Then there are all the racing thoughts in your mind, which form a kind of distracting cloud preventing you from seeing the real you. These, equally, do not need to be attached to you; let them go. You are in control of your own mind, so you do not need these thoughts. Decide which ones are useful and which ones are not, and rid your mind of any unwelcome ones.

What you have revealed in yourself will be very peaceful; for our essential nature, our spiritual self stripped of all labels and clear of all unwanted thoughts, is peaceful. At the core of our being is a deep peace. This is a journey of discovery; not an outer exploration of foreign lands but an inner journey to meet up with an old friend whom we have long forgotten.

God consciousness

What kind of relationship do you have with God? The first step towards awareness of God is the belief or experience of God's existence. Some people pray as a way of opening that communication; prayers requesting health and happiness for themselves or others; or prayers of thanks or praise. Others keep a daily journal in which they write to God, as one may write to a friend or advisor. Another way of communicating with God is through the experience of meditation, as described on page 83–4.

Collective consciousness: thinking globally, acting locally

Jennifer was a worrier, but also a lady very sensitive to the suffering of others. It really upset her to watch television reports of poverty and deprivation. Often she used to come to me with palpitations and chest aches the morning after seeing such programmes. What could she do being so open to others' hardships? It was making her ill. She decided to volunteer to work at the Oxfam charity shop in the village, finding that she consoled herself by knowing she was doing what she could to help those suffering in other countries. Simply being part of a group serving a common purpose shifted the focus of attention from herself. She was giving of herself in a selfless, loving way that seemed to put her own fears into perspective and, as a result, her symptoms lessened over a period of time.

The noise and bustle we experience at a personal level are also happening at a global level. There is constant activity, with so much energy being spent on reaching goals among groups, organisations and nations. There is a kind of global anxiety about always achieving results. There is worry about the economy, housing, poverty, even the weather. These are all legitimate concerns and complex matters, but we need to use the spiritual approach to such challenges. Recognising global concerns is the first move towards solutions. No problem is too difficult to overcome if our intentions are for the best. We each need to start in our own small way and then do what we can. From a spiritual point of view, it is not how much we give, but the intention behind the giving that is important; are we giving with hope, enthusiasm, understanding and kindness?

I mentioned earlier how worrying thoughts have energy and add to the collective fear; and also how having such loving thoughts add to the total sum of collective, positive feelings. Changing thoughts of fear to love can begin to change the world.

Spiritual qualities for worry

Calm

Calmness is a still mind
And is clarity at all levels
Calmness allows peace to come through
It means our actions are deliberate and unhurried.
Calmness creates harmony and leads to serenity.

To integrate positive spiritual qualities we need to think, feel and act these positive qualities. In the case of worry I have chosen calmness and mindfulness. It is not that easy just to think calmly when one is worried, because the very problem with worry is that the mind is constantly recycling problems. Thoughts race around out of habit, never finding a resting place. The moment one worry seems to be resolved, another appears. Start by using affirmations such as 'I am calm' or 'I am a calm person' or 'I feel totally relaxed'. If you are the sort of person who frequently gets anxious, write down such an affirmation on a piece of paper and carry it in your pocket to produce at difficult moments.

As with the exercise for anger, try to remember a situation when you were very calm and relaxed, and reconnect with that feeling; then bring that feeling into the situation which you find so worrying. Observe if anything changes.

When a patient is very anxious I find they can begin to make me twitchy and restless, so I try to imagine that I am sealed off in a blue cloud of calm. As my cloud grows, it engulfs the patient, too; the effect calms the patient as well as me.

Mindfulness

Mindfulness is emptying out waste thoughts
And filling with clarity.
Mindfulness is openness.
It has no expectations.
Mindfulness is being fully awake in the present.

When gardening, I frequently find myself thinking about work; and when at work I think about what needs to be done in the garden. I need to learn to work at work and garden in the garden, without distractions. This is true of many of the tasks I do every day; thoughts crowd in about things I can do nothing about. They are either in the past or have not yet happened. The challenge is to give our full attention to the task we are dealing with, whether it be washing the dishes, eating, walking or reading. Give your whole mind and body to the process in which you are involved and try to bring your mind into the present, away from yesterday's and tomorrow's concerns. This means to be fully accepting without taking a judgemental stance.

If we are truly in the present, we will not be worried about the past or future. This observation has been written about by many poets and philosophers over the centuries. Mindfulness is not easy and is often so different from our usual pattern of thought. In the surgery I commonly observe that when I greet patients, the majority will comment on the weather in a negative way. It is either too hot, too cold, too wet, no rain and so on. Now I try to be positive about the weather. Thinking and saying positive things creates a beneficial atmosphere. The next step is mindfulness, in which one moves away from the judgement of good or bad, but just is. If we can learn to be more accepting of everything in this way, it will prove to be a powerful antidote to worry.

THE APPLE EXERCISE

When sitting relaxed – in the way that has already been described – place an apple in front of you. Now focus your attention fully on the apple, observing every detail you can about it. Look at its shape;

how it is like a sphere but not quite, and how this apple has its own individual shape. Observe the colour on its surface, the various shades and textures and how the light affects it. Now begin to imagine biting into the apple; the moisture, the taste and how the apple will look with a bite out of it. Think of the seeds in the apple, and what happens when a seed germinates in the ground and grows into a small tree, eventually to produce apples. You can use your imagination to go on exploring the theme of the apple, but try to hold your concentration on the apple in front of you. You will at first find this exercise in concentration difficult to maintain much longer than several minutes before your mind wanders. This exercise can be repeated using a candle or any object, and is a method of improving our focused attention, or mindfulness.

Spiritual practice

When practising these spiritual exercises we must not be too critical of ourselves. There will be days – sometimes weeks – when we will forget to practise some of the exercises suggested. Be gentle with yourself; accept yourself. This in itself is good spiritual practice. Be mindful of who you are, where you have come from and where you are going. Our purpose is not to create more worries about your spiritual health to join the physical and mental worries. Return to the moment, and begin to focus on what you are doing with full attention, without distraction. This is being mindful, and is a spiritual practice in itself.

Twenty-one Tips for Overcoming Worry

1   **Think positively.** Be an optimist and look on the bright side of life.

2   **Share your problem.** Talk to someone you can trust, preferably someone not in your family.

3   **Sleep more.** Be aware when you are tired, and get enough sleep to rest and refresh yourself.

4   **Learn to say NO.** When asked to take on yet another task, politely decline.

5   **Do one job at a time.** Focus your attention on the job in front of you, and do not worry about what you have completed or what you should be doing next.

6   **Relax.** Study relaxation by buying a book on the subject, or buy a tape. There are many different types of relaxation, and one is sure to suit you.

7   **Play.** Make time to do the things that you enjoy doing.

8   **Delegate.** Offload some of your work and responsibilities on to others at work and even at home.

9   **Physical activity.** Take up a new activity such as swimming, walking, cycling or anything you enjoy. Try to fit in to your daily schedule.

10   **Acceptance.** Accept what you cannot change, and learn to 'go with the flow'.

11   **Eat regularly and slowly.** Make every meal an enjoyable event. Eat plenty of fresh fruit and vegetables. Reduce fatty food and sugar.

12   **Avoid medication.** Do try not to take tranquillisers or smoke cigarettes. Do not drink more than 3 units of alcohol per day or 3 cups of coffee.

13   **Care for yourself.** If you are ill, do not pretend that you are not.

14   **Plan.** Manage your time, and make a timetable; then do not overload it.

15   **Service.** Do something for others, and you will be rewarded more than you expect.

16   **Hobbies.** Take up a new hobby; choose something you've always wanted to do, and do it now.

17   **Make time.** Take your holiday entitlement each year. Put aside at least half a day per week to do something you want to do. Each day, schedule breaks just for peace and quiet.

18   **Commitments.** Anything that you really do not enjoy doing, give up now. They will cope without you!

19   **Realism.** Be realistic about what you consider to be perfection, and what you can achieve.

20   **Remember.** You are a person of worth. You are a unique individual with valuable qualities that are continually being developed.

21   **Smile.** Keeping a smile on your face not only makes you feel better, but it cheers up everyone else too.

Guilt

....

Guilt is a burden. It is an unnecessary load to carry, and it slows us down on our journey towards optimum health. It makes life joyless, and in common with the other negative attributes, it leads to unhappiness and illness.

Shame

The immediate experience of guilt is shame. Like a secret, it's thought if it is exposed it will lead to ridicule or condemnation. Such shame is worth while uncovering, as with all guilt there is a desperate need to share the secret.

Janice was a lady who had been a patient for fifteen years, often consulting with aches and pains which nearly always failed to respond to any treatment. The root cause was elusive. Then one day she came in to see me in a panic, as her husband said he had had enough, and demanded they sit down and get to the bottom of her problem that very afternoon. She had a terrible feeling of guilt that was constantly playing on her mind. For years she had been able to suppress it, but now it was stronger than ever and she was terrified of revealing it. Slowly, she told me that twenty years ago she had flirted with her husband's best friend at a party, and later felt so ashamed. This confession to me in the surgery made it easier for her to tell her husband later and over the next few weeks her aches and pains gradually melted away.

Sometimes such cases may seem trivial to us, but to the individual the very suppression of the shame gives it more energy and, paradoxically, saps one's physical vitality to some degree. The next case, despite his confession, was unable to forgive himself.

Andre had not been feeling himself for some years, and had recently developed chest pains when exercising. At sixty-five he wasn't particularly old for such a heart complaint and there was much that could be done to help him; but he said that the pains were something to be expected at his age and refused any further tests. At the time it struck me as an unreasonable attitude because he had achieved much in his business, and had a successful family life. Over the months his condition deteriorated, and on one occasion when I visited him at home he stated he did not wish to receive any special treatment, as he felt he did not deserve it. I paused and waited through the silence. With a deep sigh he told his story. He was studying at university in Holland at the outbreak of the Second World War. He was a keen sportsman with many friends. When the Germans invaded he escaped to stay with relatives in the outlying countryside. After the war he discovered that most of his friends, who had remained in the town, had been killed fighting for the Resistance. He felt guilty for escaping to the countryside and not joining them, and this guilt haunted him every day of his life. The love of life he had experienced with his friends as a student had been broken by the weight of his guilt. Even after this confession to me, and later to others, he was unable to forgive himself. Six months after that day he died of a heart attack.

Many patients I see where the underlying problem is guilt tend to have a 'victim' mentality: a feeling of being punished, and in addition feeling they deserve it. It often shows in what they say about themselves. Some examples are: 'I feel unworthy . . .' 'I am not good enough . . .' 'Everyone treats me like this . . .' 'I deserve this illness . . .' 'Nobody understands me . . .'

These phrases played over and over in the mind reinforce the guilt, and in turn give rise to hopeless resignation: 'I cannot help it . . . it is just the way I am . . .' 'I do not have time to . . .' 'There is no way this can change . . .' 'Nothing I do will help . . .'

All are statements of poor self-esteem where the person is no longer able to love themselves.

If such phrases are constantly repeated they become 'a mind-set'; like a record stuck in a groove, repeating the same tune over and over. There is a pay-off for the person as it can become a convenient excuse. This leads to other mind-sets: 'Nothing is my fault because of my circumstances.' 'It is not my fault, it is the way I was brought up.'

One of the most common mechanisms that hinders the opportunity to achieve optimum health is the adoption of the victim mentality. It is such mind-sets that provide the perfect excuse to avoid taking responsibility for an illness.

Blame

Guilt that can be expressed, but not acknowledged as our own, can be projected on to others by blaming them. And so there is a whole new set of mind-sets: 'She made me do . . .' 'It is his fault . . .' 'If it were not for her . . .' 'She will be sorry . . .' 'He makes me . . .' 'He hurt my feelings . . .'

Mrs Flowers was short of breath, which she told me was caused by asthma. I asked when the asthma had started, and she said as a child when her mother had left her in a damp bedroom. More allergies started after her previous doctor had given her antibiotics. She had visited various therapists, but none was able to help her, and she now did not think it worth spending any more money. Nothing could be done, and no one could help her. She was stuck in a negative thought pattern of blaming everyone, which may well have begun in childhood. Perhaps she had reason to blame someone all those years ago, but such an attitude was now no longer appropriate, and blocked her recovery.

Blame which is expressed can not only be projected on to others, but also towards ourselves. In this next example there is another mind-set phrase, 'if only'.

Mr Jackson seemed a very capable man who had looked after his disabled wife for fifteen years. He himself had now developed indigestion, and while I was examining him he took the opportunity, which he always did, to talk about his wife. She had been left paralysed on one side from a stroke, and needed a lot of nursing care at home. He blamed the nurses for not dressing his wife's leg ulcer properly, and the social worker for not providing the right equipment. Given the opportunity he blamed everyone involved in her care. Then he said she hadn't done enough, and had not been assertive enough at the hospital when she last had her ulcer attended to. He felt he should have called the doctor earlier, and if only he hadn't been so clumsy and knocked her leg in the first place. He went right back to her original accident; he was sure that he himself should have gone out to get the groceries on the night she had the stroke. If only he had done all these things differently. He was guilty of all these crimes, and now felt he was getting his due punishment by having the indigestion. In some ways he was right: his symptoms were due to him blaming himself, and perhaps he could no longer 'stomach the guilt'.

'If only I called the ambulance earlier . . .' 'If only I had listened to what he'd said . . .' 'If only the doctor had diagnosed it earlier . . . this wouldn't have happened.'

'I ought to have' is a similar expression, used when we blame ourselves for not doing our duty. It is as though we have a kind of inner figure who is critical of every move and decision we make, constantly whispering over our shoulder that we are not good enough, or could have done better.

Gossip

World-wide a favourite way of passing time is to gossip; on street corners, behind curtains, at the office – anywhere and everywhere. This kind of exchange is not productive conversation, but is the constant negative comment on the behaviour of others. Gossip may seem harmless enough, but think of the times when you have been part of it; the judgement is rarely balanced and circumstances are often exaggerated. Blame is too easily apportioned and rumours begin to spread. Gossiping can soon become a habit of being negative about others.

The chatter of idle gossip is a means of self-deception with which we avoid responsibility for our own actions by blaming others. If we criticise others what are our own shortcomings? By pointing the finger, where does our own guilt lie?

Punishment

Persistent feelings of guilt lead to the need to punish. If it is shame it is self-punishment, leading to lack of self-worth and depression. If blame of others the punishment can be violent.

Jonathan's case of self-punishment is one that I will always remember. He was only twenty-nine when he first consulted me with the lump on his back; one year later he was dead. It seemed he had everything to live for: a young son, a new job, a new house and a caring, supportive wife. His tumour turned out to be rapidly malignant and didn't respond to surgery, radiotherapy or chemotherapy. Most of his specialised treatment was carried out in hospital, and as his general practitioner I only became involved when he was sent home to die. He was given the finest hospice home-care support by a group of dedicated nurses, but his pain control with even the strongest painkillers was proving difficult. He said he would give anything for a decent night's rest. Fortunately a healer friend of mine lived nearby, and he agreed to receive some healing. The next time I visited he and his wife were delighted, as at last he had had several undisturbed nights, and even began to reduce his painkillers. However, when the pain returned he just didn't seem to want to seek relief by asking for the healer to return. At the deepest level he was tormenting himself, and despite every effort by those caring for him was unable to die peacefully.

No rational explanation could be found for why Jonathan did not want relief from his pain. When those of us caring for him discussed his case after his death we all felt intuitively that the root of his illness was guilt. Why was he punishing himself we will never know; and perhaps he was not consciously aware himself of the reason that he allowed himself to suffer the pain. He seemed to have some hidden guilt that he could not share and perhaps felt he needed to suffer to pay off his debt.

Judgement, using discrimination

It can seem obvious at first, the rights and wrongs of a given situation, but on closer inspection it can prove more difficult to decide who is to blame.

Joan knew that her symptoms – headaches, poor sleep and bad temper – were all due to her impending divorce. She was worried about the children and was finding it difficult to manage on her own. She was anxious and depressed.

Some days later her husband Duncan came to see me. He told me he was in tears most of the day, and found concentrating at work impossible. He was fearful he would lose his job if he stayed off work much longer. He was particularly upset as he had just learned that Joan had been unfaithful to him over several years.

I learned later that Duncan himself had had an affair ten years before. Who is to blame: Joan or Duncan, or is it the fault of their lovers?

Both Joan and Duncan had far from happy childhoods, as Joan's parents divorced when she was nine, and Duncan's father had a string of girlfriends he brought home when Duncan's mother was ill in hospital. They in turn must each bear some responsibility for the impending divorce between Joan and Duncan. And their behaviour in their marriage may, in turn, have been influenced by their parents before them.

Rarely do two people agree to the exact truth of a situation. Each will be influenced by their own experiences and background. They will be influenced by others' views, and be biased because of some recent event. If we are honest, much will depend on our emotional state at the time.

There is this part of us that is constantly critical of everything we do or say, like a strict schoolmaster, or a scolding parent always demanding perfection. When making this internal judgement it is usually negative, leaving the feeling of guilt. As for judging ourselves we are strict towards ourselves in a way that we would not be to others. There is no appeal court, no mitigating circumstances, and no forgiveness. It is the weight of such guilt that eventually results in physical and mental symptoms, so that in turn we expect others to live by the standards we set ourselves. The blame is now directed externally on to others.

The problem is that if we are harsh internally with ourselves it becomes a habit; so we become harsh externally with others. We become the critical friend, the strict parent, the authoritarian schoolmaster, the law-enforcing policeman.

As you may begin to realise the whole process of making a balanced judgment becomes more complex, and frankly not very reliable. However, studying how we do make judgements is the key to unlocking the chains of guilt.

We make judgements of everything and everybody on two levels. At the usual thinking level the critical appraisal goes on. This is essential to distinguish between opposites and make choices, hot and cold, black and white, good and bad. What it is not so good at is distinguishing between the rights and wrongs of moral judgements. That is done better by tapping into the deeper level of our conscience.

First is means shutting off the critical parent, teacher, or policeman in our heads, then standing back regardless of what is happening in the outer world, stilling ourselves, and looking at the bigger picture in a detached way. It is a calm appraisal free of emotions and attachment. It is listening to the inner still voice that breaks through the confusion with clarity. This is the process of discrimination at the highest and best level.

Our conscience acts like a monitor, informing us of the truth of any situation. It will be free of others' opinions, our present emotional state, and even our beliefs. It comes from a much deeper place; and it is that which informs us of the truth.

In practice, before making any decision or offering an opinion, stop and check inwardly. What is the truth? When you are sure, give your measured opinion. It will be personal, and often at odds with the general trend, but it will be your truth. If you learn to act on this you will never experience any guilt. It is when this conscience is ignored that guilt will fester, ultimately leading to illness, both physical and mental.

Besides checking inwardly with our conscience at a deeper level, we can develop a discriminating mind by choosing the thoughts on which we focus at the personality level. Take, for example, the situation of someone expressing their anger in whose firing line you happen to be. Suspend your critical mind; using your discriminatory power you can choose not to take on any of this anger, but focus instead on your own inner qualities of tolerance and understanding. This not only helps you, but also helps the person who is angry.

It is healing to take responsibility for your actions and not attribute blame to others, or fate. It is healing to say sorry when appropriate, and resolve to do better. Discriminating is not to criticise constantly, but to provide an alarm when we are not acting according to our higher nature. Being non-judgemental is an essential attitude with optimum healing.

Justice

Anyone who has had experience of law courts will understand that rarely is there a satisfactory outcome for either side. The court's job is to interpret the law, to uphold the social order, to make a judgement, and then to mete out punishment.

But there is another justice that has nothing to do with courts. It is the spiritual law of cause and effect, referred to in the East as karma. It simply means 'what we put out will come back to us in equal measure.' Any negative word, any negative thought, any negative action, will come back to us. It will return some time. We will be the recipient of what we have done to others. The same is true of any positive thought, word, or action. This 'law' is as sure as any physical law, so there is justice, a moral justice, which is weighed in each of our hearts.

Ways of dealing with guilt

Beginning to understand guilt is central to releasing it as a negative quality. These specific suggestions are made as a practical start to the healing process.

1 Changing mind-sets

We are born with the body we have, and cannot do much to change it. We cannot change our parents. We certainly need to recognise we cannot change others. But we do have the power to change our way of thinking.

However it is not that easy. The first hurdle is to recognise some of the mind-sets we may be locked into. Second, the way we think can be comfortable, and the effort to change can seem to be too much. One thing is sure: if you do have a longstanding illness you are likely to be fixed into thinking in a certain way. But the good news is if you do want to get better you can, by changing your thinking. After all, healing is about change. Easy to say, but perhaps the most difficult thing to do.

A simple method that has already been suggested in this book is to create affirmations. Examples such as, 'I am a healthy person,' or 'I will get better,' are a good start.

More specific affirmations can be very helpful for certain conditions. If you have dry itchy skin the mind-set could be, 'I have had this for years and none of the creams do any good.' The affirmation would be, 'My skin is soft and smooth, and each day the cream becomes more effective.' If you have poor eyesight you could repeat to yourself, 'My vision is improving every day.'

If you are aware what your mind-set is you can begin to work at a deeper level. Take the examples we have already given. 'If only . . .' can be replaced with 'I take responsibility for my own actions.' 'I ought to . . .' can be replaced by 'I will act according to my conscience.' 'I am useless . . .' can be replaced by 'I have many qualities which I can share with others.'

Making up your own affirmations gives them more power. You can write them down, and stick them in places where you will see them. In your diary, on the telephone, on the refrigerator door, or on your desk at work. You can say them out loud whenever you remember, or chant them fifty time a day. You are retraining your mind with new thoughts, and pushing out the old ones. If you catch yourself thinking in a negative way, replace the old pattern with a new one.

2 Counselling: sharing the secret

Some of the patients described in this chapter were able to share their distress, and discover for themselves that guilt was the underlying cause of their condition. It was the first step to seeing that optimum health is achievable. Having the courage to share a secret with someone else is often such a relief that symptoms fall away. It is best to choose someone not close to you who themselves will not form any judgement. That is why going to a trained counsellor can be so useful, but sometimes working it through on your own can be really helpful.

Sheila Jones, an English teacher, had been off work because of stress and depression for two years. She told me that she used to be such a lively person and that going to work in the morning was such a joy. Now, some days she could hardly get out of bed and seemed to be full of thoughts of doom. She had been to counselling and thought a lot about the cause of her problems. There were the deaths of two friends, and the upheavals at work contributed to her stress. She could also reflect that problems in her childhood played their part. She was stuck, and the main feeling she was left with was guilt. But why guilt? She had no idea. I suggested she might like to write her life story as a dialogue, in which she took one part and the other was taken by a helpful guide. She liked this idea and went off to write her story. She returned some months later to tell me of her progress on her autobiography. She recounted how it had been a difficult and sometimes painful exercise. Eventually she was able to write her guilty feelings as a confession. Slowly the burden of guilt was shed. She found that spark to life again, and began to enjoy herself. She never went back to teaching, and later became a secretary instead.

If you do have a guilty conscience concerning someone or something, write it down. It is a good way to confess. Even better, take a large piece of paper and list all your guilt feelings. Alongside each item write down how you could have done better, and what you will now do to change. Ultimately we are our own judges; who better to know of the sincerity of our confession? Also what good practice to be generous by forgiving ourselves!

When it comes to the actions of another who, through our conscience, we understand to be wrong, we need, rather than to criticise, to be an example. This will encourage them to take any necessary steps towards change.

3 Remorse: saying sorry and acting sorry

Remorse is when we feel guilt and sorrow at the same time. If the remorse is genuine, and demonstrable by good actions, the guilt can be absolved. This is true for even the worst of crimes. The final judgement is really one's own conscience, and it is that which informs us of what is morally right or wrong. But do not be too harsh with yourself. We do have to make choices in our lives, and that sometimes involves making the wrong one. Even if we have the right intention, things can go wrong. Say sorry for the mistake and learn from the experience. There is nothing to be gained by holding on to guilt feelings.

Ann had injured her back in a car accident two years previously, and was involved in an insurance claim against the other driver. One thing was certain: her back pain would not begin to improve until her court case was heard, and a judgement made. She was so full of blaming the other person that she could not admit that she was partly to blame. She had osteopathic manipulation as part of her treatment for her back and during her treatment recounted what had really happened. She said that just before the accident she had been tidying her hair in the car mirror, and at that moment of distraction she had crashed. The other driver whom she collided with had been driving dangerously, but her inattention had contributed to the accident. Admitting her blame to the insurance company meant that perhaps she would not get the full claim, but from that time on she made a speedy recovery.

Like the other negative qualities, the purpose of guilt may be to encourage us to change. It is not pleasant to feel guilt and shame. The approach is the same: take responsibility for your thoughts, feelings and symptoms and change your attitude. Later, emotional, mental and physical changes will follow.

Rob Blackwell had consulted me about a cough, and took the opportunity to tell me that his old hand injury was playing him up. He went on to explain that he had sustained the injury fifty years ago, shortly after the D-day landings. He was part of a tank crew, and one day on patrol asked his commander to stop so he could relieve himself. While he was behind a bush the tank received a direct hit; all his comrades were killed and from the explosion he received a shrapnel wound to his hand. He felt terrible guilt that he had asked the tank to stop, thus making it an easy target. In addition there was the guilt of being the only survivor. Through his guilt he felt a deep remorse, and over the years did what he could for the relatives of those killed. They never blamed him, but he could not rid himself of the guilt. He committed himself to a lifetime of service to others. The guilt faded over the years, but the occasional pain in his injured hand reminded him of the promise he had made to himself to be of service to others till the end of his days.

He told me that through his serving others as a kind of penance, not only did his guilty burden become lighter, but he felt more at peace within himself. This served as a deep healing for him.

4 Thinking positively

For most of us in any situation it is the habit of a lifetime to think of the negative option first. It does mean as we assess positive and negative sides we tend to focus on the negative. I always find it interesting if you ask anyone to say something positive about themselves how difficult they find it, yet how easy they find it to be critical. To change this way of thinking takes practice and determination. And where better to start than on ourselves?

Try to notice when you start thinking negatively about any issue, situation or person, including yourself; and when you do, follow such thoughts by thinking of something positive. Begin with yourself, and list all your positive features. Once you have done that add all your other attributes and skills. It is so important to see ourselves in a positive way, and not constantly criticise ourselves.

Even in the worst situation something positive can always be found. Of course we must be realistic, but look for the positive aspect. I have found this is the best way to approach patients who want to know the prognosis of a serious illness: an honest appraisal, followed by a hopeful outcome.

In our own lives, besides trying to think about being positive, we need actively to seek out what is positive. Mix with people who show positive qualities; read books and watch programmes on television that make you feel good; listen to music that you find uplifting; and visit places that give you spiritual inspiration.

5 Finding peace

The experience of the deepest part of ourselves is free of all the negative qualities, and is not weighed down by the heavy burden of guilt. As we become more familiar with this quiet place, the inner discriminatory mind will be able to be heard more readily. Choices informed by this part will fill us with confidence, and by their very nature will be free of blame.

In essence we are good. When we are not in touch with this state of peace we are not bad, we are out in the world, suffering and learning. We can be lazy and forget our true nature, but we are not bad.

We may occasionally have a sense of peace in our ordinary day. Seeing the sun rising in the morning, relaxing in a hot bath, or drifting into a pleasant daydream bring a longing for that peace. However, such moments are usually transient, and if we wish to cultivate a more lasting experience of peace we should put time aside each day to practise some of the exercises suggested already and some more specific ones for guilt.

RELEASING GUILT

First find a place that is quiet, and allow yourself some time. As described in the chapter on worry relax the body, calm the emotions and still the mind. Focus on breathing, and with your imagination . . .

. . . See yourself on a journey, perhaps along a path through a wood. It leads towards a castle. Before the path reaches the castle there is a river, with a bridge crossing it. Whatever burdens you are carrying, in terms of baggage or otherwise, leave on this side of the bridge before crossing. Now walk on towards the castle, which you enter through open gates into a large hall. Once inside, you experience a sense of peacefulness. You stand in the centre of this sacred place, and when you look up you see from an opening in the roof golden rays of the sun coming through. The sun shines as a beam of light on where you are standing and bathes your whole body. These rays of light seem to go through you, cleansing you from top to bottom. All the impurities are washed away until every cell is clean and fresh. You stand there enjoying this feeling of renewal, and stay as long as you need. When it is right, you decide to leave. You walk out of the hall through the gate out of the castle, back to the bridge. You cross over and see the burden you came with lying by the bridge. You now have a choice: to pick it up or leave the burden behind.

Slowly come back to where you are sitting holding on to the feeling of purity and lightness. Can you name what the burden was, and were you able to leave it behind? When you open your eyes sit quietly for a few minutes, and experience how you feel before returning to your normal activities.

A FORGIVING PERSON

Again when you are in a state of relaxation, using your imagination . . . see a person sitting opposite you who looks completely at peace. Think of that person as representing the highest of qualities, such as truth, humility and compassion. He or she sits looking at you with kindness and understanding. They are completely at peace, and have the qualities of patience, tolerance and wisdom. You look at the eyes; they are soft, and have a great depth to them. You feel a warmth and closeness to this person. They are the perfect person, a trusted friend and companion, loving and forgiving. You can tell them anything, and they will listen with complete under-standing. So you tell of your guilt, slowly going over in detail why you are feeling guilty. When you have finished they are still looking at you with unconditional love, and although nothing is said you know you have been forgiven.

Spiritual awareness

Soul consciousness

The kind of attitude that is healthy to develop is one of freedom from judging others and attributing blame; and judging ourselves and feeling guilt. Judgement is a function of the ego consciousness. Soul consciousness is that conscious awareness where we use the inner wisdom to solve conflicting complex issues in a discriminating way.

How can one be more soul conscious without guilt in everyday activities? Resolving to refrain from criticising others, and not partaking in gossip is a good start. In the work situation if you feel you have to criticise someone, it is good practice to stop and take a detached view. See the positive aspects of the other person first. That also means releasing the negative attribute of guilt within ourselves, which frees us to see the positive qualities in ourselves, and so we can then see them in others.

God consciousness

When you feel badly about yourself it is difficult to receive the love of others. When we are preoccupied with shame and our own misdemeanours it is difficult to be open to the universal love that comes from God. So it is important to make every effort to release any guilt we may have. Simply by learning to love ourselves we open ourselves to receive love, and if one reflects on that it is true in all our relationships.

In addition, if one has an image of God as an authoritarian figure, one can feel that one is being judged by the almighty: like a figure on a throne sitting in judgement on every action to mete out punishment. Is that really a god of love?

Mrs Shaney was frightened about the skin lumps on her back. She asked immediately if it was cancer as her husband had died of cancer two years previously. A quick look and I was able to reassure her that they were only fatty swellings. Her concern about them turned out to be an indication of her inner frame of mind. She wanted to talk; first about how she worried about her health, and then how she was sure she would be punished for her past crimes. She felt she had not done enough to care for her husband, and felt guilty that she was relieved that he had died. In addition she felt guilty for wanting to enjoy herself. Now God was punishing her for such a selfish thought. She had always been a devout Christian, but thought it wrong that God should punish her, and then felt guilty about such a thought.

As children we learn about God from our parents and what we are taught at school. The image we have of God is often a male authoritarian figure judging each action. That in turn fashions our beliefs and the way we live our life. Sooner or later that belief is tested by circumstances which seriously challenge the basis of our belief, or may even deepen it.

Jane was forty-five when her husband was killed in a car crash. It appeared to everyone she had coped very well over the years. She developed a stomach pain months after his death, and despite extensive investigations and treatments for the pains they never let up. During one consultation she described the pain as 'her burden'. I asked her what she meant. She confessed it was her punishment for blaming God for taking her husband away, and her subsequent lack of faith. At a follow-up visit she admitted that now she had shared her secret it had seemed lighter. This confession allowed her to reconsider the relationship she had with God. Was he really handing out more punishment to add to her suffering? Months later she told me that when she began to understand that God was as compassionate being and not vengeful, the stomach pains went.

Knowledge of the transcendent, which is different from belief, comes through personal experience and is often the result of suffering. With this comes a deepening of our understanding of His nature. I say His nature, but part of that understanding is that God is neither male or female, is beyond gender. This concept of 'being beyond' begins to give a sense of the experience of the absoluteness of God's nature. At this level there is no right or wrong, good or evil. There is just the absolute, as the mystics describe: a oneness with no division.

Collective consciousness

The collective consciousness is the sense of feeling a part of everything, and may not necessarily depend on a belief in God. I did distinguish between belief and knowledge: belief is something that is taught, and knowledge is gained through personal experience. When one moves into the experience of being connected to all beings, God consciousness and collective consciousness are very similar experiences.

Understanding this can be helpful when dealing with guilt. It gives the ability to see ourselves in others, and others in ourselves. The mistakes we make are mistakes that most people will have made; and likewise their mistakes are more than likely at some time to have been committed by us.

Just as we focused on individual spiritual qualities as a way of being soul conscious we can do the same in a group, by developing common values as a way of being collective conscious. For example, in our surgery our receptionists decided that their values as a group were to be friendly, co-operative and supportive of each other as a team. The staff in the office doing mainly administrative work identified their values as efficiency and caring. When a problem arises within the group the question has to be asked if such issues are helpful to the overall common positive qualities of that group. If not, the issue should be put to one side, and dealt with later. This is not to deny that such feelings or negativity are around, but at that particular time it is interfering with the group process. Often we have found that by focusing on the positive qualities of the group the interpersonal issues seem to fade away. It is not so much that we are ignoring the dark side, but that the light seems to disperse it.

Spiritual qualities for guilt: forgiveness and compassion

In each of the chapters on the negative attributes I have chosen their opposite positive qualities, and you may wish to choose those which to you are more appropriate. For anger, I chose tolerance and patience; for depression, hope and enthusiasm; for worry, calmness and mindfulness; and for attachment; generosity and humility. When the root problem is guilt I have chosen forgiveness and compassion.

Forgiveness

Forgiveness is letting go of blame and guilt.
And it lightens the load
Forgiveness is simple,
It is not easy.
Forgiveness makes the way clearer.

Forgiveness is not something that comes easily to a lot of people. We may feel sure about what is right and wrong, but who is sure enough to judge another, and to punish the crime? The spiritual approach is not one of blame but of understanding that, given the same circumstances, we are capable of acting in the same way. It is to act with the gentleness one would show to a child learning to walk, encouragement of success, an easiness with failure.

FORGIVING OURSELVES

We can only learn to forgive others if we can first learn to forgive ourselves. It takes repeated practice, and do not be harsh on yourself. Be gentle. You may have made a mistake, or committed a crime, but there is nothing to be gained from holding on to the guilt endlessly. Learn from your experience and resolve to improve. Only that way can you make progress towards optimum health, and prevent the burden of guilt showing itself as an illness. Recognise it, admit it, and express your sorrow.

FORGIVING OTHERS

However badly you feel someone has treated you, you must eventually forgive them. Blaming others and holding on to hate will only diminish you yourself. As we know, negative feelings of revenge and anger lead to illness. They serve no purpose in those on the healing path.

Forgiveness is understanding that we too are guilty. In any unpleasant situation we have to begin to understand that we also played a part. The other was not wholly to blame and we must take some of the responsibility.

Seeing some good in those who have wronged us takes great courage, especially if we think of the horrors of such crimes of torture, rape and murder. We have to move away from the view of perpetrators of such crimes as totally evil. We do not have to change our views of the crimes themselves, or of the social consequences of such crimes, but learn to see that the person committing them has potential for good. We need to relate to that goodness so we have a more balanced opinion; and that frees us from the deep-seated negative feelings of hate, revenge and anger.

When we read of crimes in other towns or countries, we need to ask if there is any way, however small, in which we played a part. We are all part of the whole and if something has happened to any part of the whole we must have contributed. Perhaps by purchasing goods from a particular country and so supporting a corrupt regime, or by not disapproving of behaviour that led to a crime. The purpose is not to pile on more guilt but to examine the situation, and if we accept that perhaps we did play a small part, we could then make a small change in ourselves. This crucial change in attitude means that when we think of the situation we are not repetitively fixed on disapproving thoughts and blame, but are looking for creative and positive solutions.

EXERCISE

In your mind's eye picture someone you blame for something they have done. Allow yourself to experience the old feelings of judgement and blame. Now detach yourself from the situation and view it from a place of love and peacefulness. Send and engulf them with the true feeling of forgiveness.

EXERCISE

Picture yourself and the other as two human beings caught up in a situation where you are wronged. Detach yourself so you can view the scene without being involved. Accept that that is how it was. Now decide and create how you would have preferred the scene to have evolved. You need to be working towards a positive outcome, without any harm to any participant.

Such exercises are very individual and are not easy, but can be repeated with different outcomes until you feel you have found a solution that leaves you free of any negative qualities and at peace. If you can manage truly to achieve this it becomes very powerful because the negative has been transformed into the positive.

ASKING FOR FORGIVENESS

If you have wronged someone and feel you need forgiveness, first apologise mentally. Picture this apology in your mind, or even say it out loud. Practise until you feel you have got it right. When you come to approach the person they will sense your good intentions. The words of apology then come easier, and are better received.

Compassion

Compassion is unconditional love.
And is thinking and acting positively.
Compassion is understanding
It is kindness and tenderness.
Compassion is the queen of qualities.

I have left compassion until last, but its importance is such that it should be at the beginning and in the middle too! It is not just a spiritual quality, it is *the* spiritual quality. Of all the qualities, compassion is the most powerful; and all the other positive qualities derive from compassion. Compassion is at the root; it is the source.

When the spiritual diagnosis is guilt, compassion is particularly appropriate, for part of the problem is a lack of love of the self. There is a reluctance by the person suffering from the guilt to believe that they are important. Such blame leads to poor self-esteem and feelings of worthlessness. If we do not accept that we have negative qualities and overcome them with love, we cannot begin to love others.

The fact remains that we cannot begin to love others if we do not first love ourselves. We need to become our own best friend, and treat ourselves with kindness and consideration; give ourselves special treats. This is not the same as being selfish or greedy; it is respecting ourselves.

Nine steps towards overcoming guilt

1   Discard the critical mind and adopt a discriminating mind.

2   Change mind-sets.

3   Counselling: sharing the secret.

4   Remorse: saying sorry and acting sorry.

5   Think positively.

6   Find peace.

7   Spiritual awareness.

8   Spiritual qualities: forgiveness and compassion.

9   Do not be harsh on yourself.

PART TWO

The first part of this book took each of the negative attributes in turn, and looked at ways of how to release them. Each had its own energy and ways of affecting us. Anger raised our energy up, whereas depression drained the energy away. Worry shakes that energy about. Attachment restricts the energy expanding and guilt holds it back.

The approach was a healing one, understanding and looking for meaning in each of the negative attributes. Seeing our goal not as one of cure, but of finding peace and developing spiritually. And finally using positive qualities as our helpers on this journey.

The second part discusses that most powerful of all the negative qualities: fear. There are five fears, and again a chapter will be devoted to discussing each one in turn. To remind you, these are the fear of: illness, accidents, change, old age and death. The most beneficial approach is to confront these fears and see them as challenges. First we must look for an understanding of each fear, and then search for meaning. The goals of optimum healing are the same, and that is to find peace and develop spiritually within ourselves.

Illness

The spiritual approach to illness is simply that the healing is in the illness itself. The human body is a self-regulating organism, with a guiding inner wisdom. When things start going wrong minor symptoms appear to warn us, and if ignored an illness will develop.

Very few people have escaped an illness of some kind or another, and everyone has had symptoms causing personal discomfort. Illness is usually seen as an interruption to our normal life that carries symptoms to be got rid of as soon as possible. Minor illness can be considered an embarrassment, and serious illness as a failure.

There are three common misunderstandings about illness. The first is not accepting one is ill in the first place. The second is trying to avoid the suffering by ignoring the symptoms in the hope that they will go away. The third is not facing the fear of illness.

Acceptance: when it is OK not to be OK

We notice time and again that people who make an appointment to see their doctor will often begin to feel better once they make an appointment, and their symptoms will miraculously improve. Like the toothache that goes when you visit the dentist. The explanation is that after a period of indecision they have accepted that they are ill and decided to do something about it.

Joyce Fox complained of a sudden onset of breathlessness two days prior to seeing me in the surgery. Despite her age of seventy-six she had always kept very fit, doing her own housework and shopping, and looking after her rather frail husband. After examining her I was able to tell her that the problem was an irregular heart rate with fluid in her lungs, probably as a result of a heart attack. A few weeks' rest at home, and taking some regular medication would normally result in a good recovery.

When I examined her at subsequent visits her clinical symptoms had improved considerably, but she continued to complain of feeling tired and suffering from palpitations. Some months passed and she was still not right, and in many ways was now worse. She was sleeping poorly at night, found difficulty concentrating, and was agitated. Before all this trouble she had always been a very active and level-headed person.

Fortunately we were running some relaxation classes at our surgery on a weekly basis, and she agreed to attend them. Over the weeks she began to improve, and when I saw her at her next review I asked her how she was. She told me she felt very much better, and felt the turning point had been when the leader of her relaxation group had talked about learning to accept the things that we cannot change. She had found it difficult to accept that she was getting older and that her illness had resulted in limitations in her ability to look after herself and her husband.

The acceptance of being ill is absolutely critical in the first step to getting better. This getting better is not just in the physical sense, but is the total well-being of the individual. The change in attitude of Joyce Fox was the change required at the spiritual level for her to begin to take that road towards her wholeness. Over the months her anxiety symptoms improved. Her feeling of tiredness, and the irregular heart rate persisted, but seemed to trouble her less. Also she and her husband became closer, because they now supported each other, whereas before she spent a lot of time caring for him.

Suffering: holding the pain

Having accepted one is ill, it is not just then a matter of looking for a cure. One has to experience the symptoms fully. The pain, the disability, the inconvenience, all have to be not only accepted, but suffered. Too many people reach for a pill to alleviate the symptoms before even considering why they are ill in the first place. If this step is missed out they will never recover. They may be cured of their symptoms, but they will not be healed.

realised this myself in a small way several years ago when I had influenza. I experienced intense muscle ache, had lost my appetite, could not concentrate, and was uncomfortable with a fluctuating fever. I lay for several days in bed suffering the discomfort, and did not even have the energy to think about getting better. It was then I decided just to give in to the illness.

My first thought was, what a relief to be off work. There was something satisfying about not having to think and make decisions. Although on a physical level I was quite uncomfortable, I had time to think. I really appreciated the peacefulness of the house while the rest of the family was out. The suffering, and giving in to the illness were necessary steps before I could begin my recovery and helped me to get over it quicker than I would have done if I'd resisted it.

I have talked to many people since who have had a similar experience with illnesses more serious than flu. With each illness we need to experience fully the symptoms and reflect why we are ill. The illness is needed at some level, and later many people say they are grateful because it prompted them to re-examine their life.

One concern I have is that modern drugs shorten or even eliminate the experience of suffering. Some people resort to painkillers too readily before asking themselves why they have the pain. Antibiotics are turned to at the first sign of infection, when in the majority of cases the body's own defences can cope adequately.

A case in point is the changing treatment of duodenal ulcers. Twenty-five years ago the choice of treatment was surgery, or six weeks' bed rest and regular meals. Both treatments worked, but many patients opted for the surgery because they got better quicker. However those who chose bed rest and a regular diet had plenty of time to reflect on why they had an ulcer in the first place. They would discover that ulcers are brought on by stress, smoking, irregular meals, and excess alcohol. The causes of duodenal ulcers are the same today, but we now prescribe a drug rather than suggest bed rest. The symptoms go within a few days, but the underlying cause is not dealt with. The result is the patient does not change, and later on they either relapse with a further ulcer, or the imbalance will show itself in some other illness.

Reflection

Illness can be a very isolating experience, and is a time for thinking. This withdrawal and inward-looking can be taken as an opportunity. A chance to ask why you're ill, and why at this time. I have seen many men in their early fifties who have had a life-threatening illness, and on recovering resolve to change their whole lifestyle completely. They all look back on their illness as something quite positive.

Try it yourself next time you have a headache, or similar minor symptom. Before reaching for the paracetamol first experience the pain and ask yourself:

> *Where is the discomfort and how would you describe it?*
> *How does it make you feel?*
> *What does it stop you doing?*
> *What lesson is it trying to teach you?*
> *How can you change to stop it happening again?*

When I had flu I considered the questions listed above, and tried to find answers. I did not find it easy, and some of the answers I came up with were quite revealing. In my case I was doing all sorts of activities too franti-cally and the illness was telling me to stop now. I learned the world went on quite well without me, and most of the tasks that seemed urgent could wait. I think the fever was the release of toxins partly related to my eating habits, and not giving time to release negativity that I had picked up during the day. I resolved to drink less coffee, and have a quiet meditation each evening.

After four to five days I knew it was time to start thinking about getting better. A week later I had recovered from the flu. I felt completely refreshed. I had not fought the illness, but surrendered to it.

Fear: facing the challenge

Fear is often quite simply due to ignorance. It is not knowing what the true facts are. Perhaps you are frightened after reading a scare-mongering article in a magazine, or listening to a neighbour who knows all about what is wrong. Equally it can be your own fantasies about the illness. Is it cancer, brain disease, and so on? Very often such fear can be overcome with just some simple information.

Mr Anderson at the age of sixty-eight developed a growth on his face, and when he learned it was cancerous he became very worried and frightened. I was able to explain to him that with his type of cancer a complete cure is nearly always achieved. He was reassured, and radiotherapy was completely successful. There would be time enough later to talk about his cancer if it was appropriate.

Cancer is not the only disease that elicits fear. Fifty years ago tuberculosis caused the same degree of fear as there was no cure then. Other illnesses have their own fears: the fear of arthritis causing disability; the fear of meningitis in children because of its sudden random nature, the fear of Aids as it strikes down young adults.

The illness is not an enemy to be fought but a challenge that has to be accepted. Suffering itself is a kind of testing, or tempering of our whole being. When we come through it there is resilience and strength.

Personality types and illness

It does seem that certain personality types develop particular illnesses. The man with the duodenal ulcer tends to be hungry for success, takes irregular nourishment, suppresses stress and ignores advice. Migraine headache sufferers are often obsessional, inflexible and rather serious. Irritable bowel syndrome sufferers are worriers and introverted.

Cancer types The basic characteristics of people who develop cancer is that they find it very difficult to love themselves. As a consequence they focus on negative qualities. Thus they feel inferior, easily feel guilty, and become depressed. The cancer personality type is emotionally repressed, especially with expressing anger. They feel they can only gain worth by taking care of others, and so are full of self-sacrifice. They tend to be martyrs, are conscientious, responsible and conform. They see life as a struggle rather than a quest for happiness.

Mrs George feared that she might develop breast cancer like her two elder sisters and her mother. It was fear that was making her ill. She had constant headaches and felt exhausted most of the time. Her children seemed always to be coming in with minor complaints. When she was young it was not done to show one's emotions and everyone had to be well-mannered at all times. Mrs George brought up her family in the same way, but it had caused quite a lot of friction between her husband and herself. He was a much more volatile and open personality. She agreed to see a counsellor, and she became more assertive and able to express her emotions. It was a long process but her relationship with her husband became more vibrant, and the children seemed to thrive. She had broken out of the family pattern of being the martyr, and probably ended the family tradition of developing cancer.

Heart attack types It has been well known that Type A personalities are more likely to develop heart disease. They are competitive and aggressive, and tend to have a chronic negative outlook. They may not be overtly hostile, but adopt a cynical approach to issues. They see life as a matter of achieving certain goals, often at the expense of other aspects of their life, and indeed other people.

These are only broad observations, and it is foolish to think that the great diversity of human beings and their illnesses can be fitted neatly into personality categories. When we describe a personality of a certain disease group such as cancer, it does not mean their personality is fixed and they cannot change. There may have been strong influences in their early years learned from parents that contribute to the way they behave. But attitudes can change, indeed need to change to prevent these illnesses developing. As a bonus, if they can bring about change they not only heal themselves, but it helps to heal other members of their own family and the members of the family that they were brought up in.

1 The meaning of illness. Is there any?

To begin to understand illness at a much deeper level we need to go beyond the idea of illness as a simple malfunction of our body. The spiritual view is that illness is a necessary part of our life, it is a challenge, and it has meaning. The desired outcome is not necessarily cure, but healing.

Doctors make a diagnosis so they can choose a rational treatment. They will also want to find a cause to the illness. The cause may be bacteria, a virus, a degenerative condition, an injury, or malfunction of an organ. In some cases one can identify psychological and social causes. This is the basis of modern medicine and generally works well at a functional level within the biomedical model.

However, it is important to distinguish between cause and meaning.

A **local town counsellor** had developed headaches with a painful neck. He wanted some quick relief as he had some important meetings to attend to, and asked for some strong painkillers. Several weeks later he returned saying although the tablets had helped they had not cured him.

Something had to be done, and be more effective this time. I suggested some physiotherapy, and after six sessions he came back saying he wished to see an orthopaedic surgeon in order to get his problem sorted out properly. Against his better judgement the surgeon operated on a vertebral disc, and somehow we all knew that it would not help this demanding man. Indeed, the headaches continued.

The town counsellor fixed on the idea that if he could just find the physical cause he would be able to put it right and get on with his life. Yet if he had reflected on his symptoms he could have discovered some meaning to them. That may have opened the door to his healing.

A danger when only looking for a cause and not meaning can lead to a sense of blame. It was someone or something's fault, and that tends to close the door on any further questioning. 'My cold was caused by someone sneezing over me.' With that attitude there is a need to ask why only you have the cold when everyone else does not.

Yet by questioning a little more you may gain a sense of why you are ill. Then you move from cause and cure to meaning and healing.

Mrs Young's catarrh had been present since she moved to her retirement house five years previously. She thought it was brought on by an allergy to the yew trees at the back of her house. When I asked her why she thought this she said the trees made her feel blocked in. She went on to say this is how she felt about living in her house. She wanted to move away, but there was no possibility because of financial reasons. It was something she was resigned to putting up with. I prescribed some nasal sprays but her blocked-up feeling never really improved.

The cause may well have been an allergy to the yew trees, but I suspect that if they were cut down she would develop further similar symptoms. The meaning of the allergy was far more likely to do with her feeling blocked in her life situation.

The function of illness is purely corrective; it is neither vindictive nor cruel. It is a means to point out, in a literal way, our own faults. Illness is to hinder us from doing more harm to ourselves, and if the symptoms are ignored they inevitably become worse.

Mr Winter was head of the language department at the local comprehensive school. It was usual for him at the end of each school term to develop some form of illness. A cold, stiff neck, or backache were his usual symptoms. However in recent years I noticed that he was taking longer than usual to recover from such episodes. He took great pride in his work and achievements, and would work most evenings and weekends. As a result his home life suffered. He always listened with respect to my suggestions, but did nothing about them. Unfortunately at the age of forty-five he had a heart attack which left him with chest pains on exercise. As a result he was unable to return to teaching, and had to reappraise his life drastically.

The symptoms were trying to show him that he needed to change the balance of his life, and when he ignored them, they eventually forced him to listen. At the spiritual level the illness was bringing to his attention the path he had strayed from.

Illness as a metaphor

The illness alerts us to the underlying disharmony and the need to change. The illness itself acts as a metaphor. It not only gives us possible insights as to why we are ill, but also reveals meaning to enable us to identify changes we need to make in order to get better.

Mrs Williams said herself the hoarseness started shortly after her husband's death. When I asked if she saw any connection, she felt it could be due to ongoing worry about the settlement of the will. She went on to explain that the problem was that her husband had argued with his sister the year before his death. He had forbidden her to talk to his sister. She now suffered the tension of wanting to fulfil her dead husband's wish, and wishing to make up with her sister-in-law. I saw her again a month later and she told me she had decided to meet her sister-in-law. They had got on famously, and had decided to go off on holiday together. The hoarseness cleared. The symptom of hoarseness was symbolic of her inability to talk about her dilemma.

The meaning of symptoms

A person will reveal much about themselves through their body posture. For example a person who sits when talking to you with arms and legs crossed does not really want to communicate with you. Whereas someone who sits leaning forward looking you in the eye is interested in what you are saying. The way we walk, the way we talk, the way we dress, all say something about who we are and how we are. What is less well accepted is that the symptoms of illness suggest why we are ill in the first place.

The interesting thing is that the symptoms we produce are very specific to each one of us, in a literal sense. The words we use give clues to the underlying meaning of the illness. If we have a discomfort in our chest and we as an individual attribute it to indigestion, it will literally mean we have difficulty digesting something or someone in our life. Whereas someone with a similar pain who thinks it's due to their heart may have problems associated with the heart, the organ we associate with love. Backache may mean at some level you are carrying too heavy a load, and a painful anus may reveal you can be 'a pain in the bum'.

Mrs Henry's bad back started after her husband's death. She explained that her backache got worse with all the tasks she had to do. It was too difficult to do everything on her own. She felt she was 'carrying the load' alone since her husband's death. Arranging some practical help for her not only eased her load physically, but let her share her burden at the spiritual level.

That illness is a metaphor for our problems is something I learned myself when I had neck pains.

had been cutting a hedge in the garden and at first I put the muscular ache down to that. But after a week it became worse and I tried to think of all the things it could be. Driving the car, poor posture when sitting, or mountain biking were all reasonable explanations. Eventually I went to have a massage. (Like most doctors I reluctantly seek help!) It was only when I was on the couch that I realised just how tense I was. It was wonderfully relaxing. Then out of my thoughts I saw an image of a rhinoceros trying to escape from my shoulders.

Such images that occur in deep relaxation are like dream images, and have a personal meaning to the dreamer. The images are symbolic. Like any symbol the meaning can be elusive, and with several layers to the meaning. Perhaps it meant I am thick-skinned and impulsive, charging blindly into things and my neck pain was a symptom of this. I also experienced a sense of wonder, with a source of untapped power. The very search for the meaning itself is healing. It brings a purpose, and with that a dignity to the person's illness. It is not to be fought and overcome, but understood.

ennifer described in some detail the cravings she had for certain types of food. This was then followed by gripping abdominal pains. She had no other complaints, and further questioning did not seem to throw any light on the cause. I had no clue as to any diagnosis, so I asked her when the problem first started. She remembered that the pains began while at work over a year ago. I asked if there was a pattern to the cravings for food, and she replied that she noticed when her friend at work was on holiday the cravings did not occur. She paused momentarily, and I think she surprised herself by her reply. After a further pause she said it was perhaps because she was jealous of her friend. She went on to say that at first she admired her friend's ability to be popular at work because of her easy smile and generous nature. The more Jennifer herself tried to be popular the more people seemed to shun her. As a result she became gripped with envy. The penny dropped, she could see how the words explained her craving and pain, and the symptoms expressed her feelings. Having realised this, she was ashamed of being so envious and selfish, and was quite resolved to make amends. Needless to say her cravings and abdominal pains settled quickly.

Finally, sometimes we are faced with an illness personally, where, try as we might, there appears to be no possible meaning. If that is the case we must not close our minds, but go on searching. This is our spiritual quest, to bring meaning to our very existence, and just because we cannot find an answer does not mean there is not one.

2 Peacefulness

Peacefulness helps when you are ill, peacefulness prevents illness, and peacefulness is the ultimate goal when recovering from an illness.

Developing this peacefulness is a useful tool to help us deal with illness when it arises. Making space in the inner world of tumbling thoughts will allow that quiet voice to be heard. It is a whisper that suggests possibilities. It points you in the direction of answers to the questions of why you are ill, and what you need to do to recover.

However it is difficult to try to develop peacefulness when we are ill, and is something to turn to for nourishment in times of need. That is why we should waste no time and begin practising now, because we receive the double benefit of it helping when we are ill and helping to prevent illness.

How then do we connect with inner peacefulness, so it is part of our daily life? First through what we do, say and think. Simply acting in a non-violent, co-operative way. Speaking only positive and peaceful words. Thinking peaceful thoughts and ideas.

Second, remembering peaceful places we have visited will help reconnect with our inner peace. A walk in the hills, the fragrance of a garden, or a swim in a lake may evoke that memory. Holding these experiences resonates with our own peacefulness. Seeking out such experiences, and then taking them in develops the peacefulness.

Third, practising some of the visualisation exercises and meditation help to expand that space in our mind that is peaceful.

3 Spiritual awareness

We are all on a spiritual journey, and illness is one of the lessons on that journey that helps us to deepen our spiritual awareness. It helps us to grow spiritually.

Soul consciousness

Illness, and the suffering it brings, often force us to focus on where the suffering is. What part of me is suffering? Is it me the personality, or is there part of me that is separate and is not suffering?

That other separate part is simpler and clearer. It does not have the distractions of the personality, and the five negative qualities. It is free of emotions and confusing thoughts. Illness draws to our attention that something is out of balance, and that we have to review what has gone wrong. This is when we need to turn inwards to get in touch with the soul level again.

At this level we can watch in a detached way the ups and downs of life much in the manner that we watch the days and seasons pass. We can be fully mindful of the present, and at the same time know that it will pass. There is an awareness in us that goes beyond the physical, emotional and mental boundaries. The soul is part of our limitless existence.

In each chapter on the treatment of negative attributes some suggestions enabling us to connect with this soul level have been made; and in particular the practice of meditation.

One may read it and think it is a good idea, but when do you think you will begin to put it into practice? I can say that of all the preventative health measures I think practising peacefulness is the most useful. If you do develop an illness it is the most helpful tool to aid to your recovery.

God consciousness

Some people have no belief in a God, while for others the understanding of God is a very personal view as to what sort of being He is.

Mrs Parkways, when attending her mother dying of a terminal cancer, called out in anguish, 'Please, God, I will suffer anything myself, but please do not let her die in pain.' The following year she developed a painful and progressive condition of her legs. She felt it was her punishment for tempting God, and she deserved the condition she now had.

Mrs Parkways does not see her God as the God of love, but as a vengeful father. She really did believe she had to accept her fate of taking God's punishment. I told her my view that a loving parent would not punish a child, and would be only too ready to forgive her. It was a view that would involve a huge step for her, but by mentioning it, it would give her something to think over.

So I believe when we make a connection with the supreme soul, it is the experience of a caring friend who gives us love unconditionally, not a harsh picture of God that we may have learned from books.

The practical ways already outlined of making that connection to experience God are meditation, prayer, contemplation, breathing in beauty.

Collective consciousness

Being ill not only affects the individual, but has implications for the immediate family and even society at large. One only has to consider a patient who suffers severe back pain and has to take to bed. It creates extra work for his wife, and may have implications for the rest of the family because of loss of income. There will be changes in the interactions within the family. The wider implications are that people at work will have to adapt to the individual being sick, and that may affect the company profits which in turn has an effect on the national economy. As it happens, many millions of hours at work are lost through back problems.

Sometimes we need to go beyond the individual to find meaning in illness. A child born with a disability such as Down's Syndrome may be thought of as having a miserable existence, and being a burden on the family. But we can look at the many positive qualities such children possess. Down's Syndrome children can be very open, friendly, and quite uninhibited. Such qualities are certainly much needed in society and in each of us. Therefore in the context of the family and people caring for them, they add something of value to the life of the group. They make a real contribution.

Many children who die young from disabling illness often give something very special to the members of their family. In the family context there is meaning in their illness. They often possess special qualities that will later remind us of them, such as courage, fearlessness, humour and willpower. Their memory encourages us to develop these positive qualities in ourselves.

We may also observe in people deprived of one of their senses the development of another to extraordinary capacity. I do not mean that they develop a compensatory sensory capacity. Blind people not only develop acute hearing, but are sensitive listeners. They develop spiritual qualities, and as a result gain in wisdom.

Sadly, a sickness in an individual can reflect a sickness in society. We only have to look at developing countries to see the result of malnutrition devastating communities. One of the main causes of such malnutrition is civil strife. Nature can always provide for man's needs, but not his greed. It is the greed of the few that results in the illness of the many. It is the negative qualities in some that lead to the disease in many.

Spiritual qualities

Willpower

Perhaps the single most desirable quality in overcoming an illness, after fully understanding the illness through acceptance, suffering and confronting fear, is the quality of willpower.

Willpower is calling on inner reserves
And bringing it into action.
Willpower is determination, and discipline.
It can move mountains.
Willpower is willingness to change.

I work in a rehabilitation unit and all the therapists comment on this being the quality that is most important for a patient to make a good recovery. They say it is not the amount of disability that determines a patient's chance of returning to an active life at home, it is their willpower. Patients who are well motivated simply progress best, regardless of all the other factors. Willpower is more important than their degree of disability, or even support at home. This willingness to try is so important even in the most difficult and complex cases.

The willingness to change is equally important. If you think about it, a certain pattern of behaviour and attitude will have led to the illness in the first place. If you want to be well, you really must be willing to change.

Courage

> Courage is strength and perseverance,
> And it inspires others.
> Courage is the companion of change.
> It requires energy and decisiveness.
> Courage is the trust to be truly oneself.

To be able to change takes real courage. To admit that you are wrong, then to take the initiative to change and carry it through to the conclusion. That takes courage.

Mrs Dixon was extremely embarrassed when recounting her story. Since the birth of her last child four years ago her husband had assaulted her when he was drunk. She was confused, upset, and felt completely helpless. If she did confront him the next day he would say he was sorry, but it would be repeated. She wanted to help him, but she did not know how, and frankly felt very antagonistic towards him. She kept her secret until three months previously when she shared the experience with her best friend, who encouraged her to seek help. It was very courageous of her to share her problem, and to try to find a solution.

We worked out a strategy to deal with the attacks where she would wake up and put on the light, stating quite explicitly that this was unacceptable. She would tell him her friend and the doctor knew of his behaviour, and she would be reporting back to them.

I was surprised to see Mr Dixon at my surgery the following day. He was a very presentable man, and immediately said he had a problem and wanted help. He was ashamed, was at a loss with himself, and wanted to save his marriage, and not split up his family. He suggested he would see a counsellor. That in its way took great courage, as he found the counselling sessions difficult. There were many issues he had to deal with arising from a very unhappy childhood. Later on he was able to enter joint counselling with his wife, and worked through problems which enabled them to stay together.

It takes courage to face up to physical difficulties such as pain and disabilities, but can take equal courage to face long-suppressed negative qualities. These may niggle away for years without one being consciously aware of them. This is what Mr Dixon had to do, to face up to the repressed anger and guilt from his childhood, and work at current problems in his relationships. It saved his marriage, and ensured a much healthier environment for his children to grow up in.

Blocks to recovery

There are three aspects I have covered in understanding illness before embarking on a recovery programme: acceptance, suffering and facing the fear. Looking for meaning can be the key that unlocks the root of the illness, and the qualities of willpower and courage are the qualities that help you on your way. But there is one other thing to consider that, unless addressed, can block the whole recovery process, and that is lack of motivation to get better.

Karen was nineteen years old, had started smoking at fifteen and now smoked twenty cigarettes per day. She had a hacking cough following a cold and it was keeping her awake at night. She was concerned that it had lasted longer than usual, and now she had a yellow sputum. I examined her chest and throat and could find no signs of a serious infection. She asked if she could have an antibiotic to clear it up, as she wanted to go to a party the following night. She had no intention of stopping smoking in the immediate future, and no motivation to make any real change. I explained that really that would not help her recovery, and the main reason the cough persisted was that her breathing tubes' lining had been damaged because of the smoking.

This is not to suggest that all smokers should be refused antibiotics, and similarly everyone with stomach ulcers withheld modern drugs. Each case has to be treated individually. But if treatment is only directed at a physical level, it will only cure that episode of illness at the physical level, and the symptoms will either recur at a later date, or become manifest of the illness at the physical level, and the symptoms will either recur at a later date, or become manifest somewhere else as another illness. To bring about healing the problem has to be tackled at a spiritual level. The illness has to be suffered, and there has to be an understanding that the illness has a meaning. The person has then to make some change such as giving up smoking, changing their diet, or altering work patterns. To do this one needs to be motivated, which requires willpower and often courage.

The five negative attributes lead to illness, but complacency prevents recovery. The lack of motivation of complacency runs deep, and although may simply appear to be laziness, at a deeper level is the unwillingness to take responsibility.

It is one of the most difficult problems that a doctor encounters when trying to help a patient help themselves. Typically, such a patient appears disinterested, cannot be bothered, or won't make any effort. Any excuse to avoid taking responsibility. The illness is an unwanted interference in their life, and they have had nothing to do with its development. It bears no relationship to their own behaviour or attitudes in the past. It is someone's fault, and the illness itself is a meaningless annoyance. 'Please, doctor, give me something to get rid of it quick.'

Perhaps such an attitude has been encouraged by doctors adopting an authoritarian manner. In turn patients are all too willing to comply.

John was thirty-five when he fell twenty feet off a scaffold and injured his back. That was ten years ago and now he was in a wheelchair. In the early years he had a lot of treatment to help with his rehabilitation, and I am sure he enjoyed the attention at the time. He always seemed a very good patient but when any progress was made there would always be some excuse not to attend the therapy. His medical notes were full of investigations. The specialists he attended were puzzled why he was not walking as there were no obvious physical reasons for this. Gradually over the years John's complacency affected those helping him, and he seemed resigned to a life in a wheelchair.

Complacency is worse in patients who have an investment in remaining unwell. The illness may have brought about sympathy and attention, and now they are unwilling to lose the role they have made for themselves. This may seem all very obvious, but such games can go on at subtle levels where the patient and carer are no longer consciously aware of what is happening. Nothing done helps, and any suggestion will be strongly resisted. If you can reassure them that the love and support will still be there when their symptoms go they may begin to recover. Unfortunately the pattern has often gone on for years and they often remain resistant to any intervention.

An aid to recovery

A useful question to ask when planning your recovery is: 'What have been the positive aspects of my illness?' It may seem rather odd to think that in suffering there could be anything good or positive. Pain, nausea, discomfort and disability are all fairly negative experiences, and you may well wonder what could possibly be positive about any of them.

Personally I do not know of any illness or disease where there is not something that is positive. The positive aspects may not be an improvement in physical symptoms, or psychological well-being, but hold spiritual lessons for our own benefit.

My own memories of childhood illness were very positive. Although I contracted the usual infectious diseases, whose symptoms can be rather unpleasant, my memory of them is quite blissful. When my brother or I became ill we would be carried through to my parents' large bed, and the fire in the bedroom would be lit. My father would buy us comics and lemonade, and we would be given little gifts to cheer us up. I remember the atmosphere in the bedroom was peaceful, and I can remember the view through the window looking over a small park. My memory of illness was the loving concern of my parents which made the physical discomfort easy to bear.

Visualise your recovery

Throughout this book different visualisation exercises have been suggested to overcome some of the negative qualities that are at the root of disease. Such visualisations are useful tools to aid recovery. The power of this image work is not to be underestimated.

Before thinking of suitable visualisations it is best to get a real feel of the illness you have. That is why when understanding an illness it is important to accept the illness, suffer it and face the fear. Where is it, and how do you feel it? Not only the symptoms, but the illness itself. Using colours, shapes, textures to describe it helps to create this thing called illness you are dealing with. Likening it to an animal can be helpful. Then, when you have a real sense of what this illness means to you, and what it is doing to you, begin to think of ways to overcome it.

Janice who had leukaemia saw the blood cells as an infestation of white ants. She felt unclean and invaded by these creatures that were attacking her own helpless cells and they would eventually eat up every organ of her body. In her imagination she saw the chemotherapy as a way of poisoning the ants, and buying her time. Then her own defending cells could get organised and strengthen themselves to repel these foreign invaders. With each ant that her cells devoured they gained in strength.

Seeing the leukemia in this way certainly helped Janice face her illness but, as a general rule of visualisation, aggressive methods are not so effective as images that are loving.

One old lady felt repulsed by the growth in her breast cancer which was so advanced that surgical removal would not help. She saw it as a black crab, and at first was very angry and resentful at having this cancer. She began to talk to this crab, and demand it leave her. She swore and cursed it for being there at this time in her life.

Nothing changed until she changed and began to talk to this crab and ask why it was there and what it was doing. She later said she learned a lot from her crab, as she now called the cancer. The tumour did not grow after that, and when she did die some years later it was not from the tumour.

Seventeen rules if you are ill

1   Accept that you are ill.

2   Do not feel guilty that you are ill.

3   You are important.

4   Take time off/out.

5   Go to bed for peace and quiet.

6   Relax, recuperate, spoil yourself.

7   Reflect on why you are ill now.

8   Listen to your body. If it says rest, then rest; if it says don't eat, then don't eat; and if it says sleep, then sleep.

9   Respond to people's concern about you, and enjoy being cared for.

10   They can manage at work without you.

11   They can manage at home without you.

12   Call on a neighbour or friend to help; most people like to be of service.

13   Think about what you can do to prevent future illness.

14   When you begin to feel better imagine yourself in full health.

15   When you are better have another day off doing something you enjoy before returning to work.

16   Remember to thank everyone who has helped while you have been ill.

17   If there have been problems at home or work because of your illness you could make suggestions for how best to deal with the situation if it happens again.

Change

Everything in the world is constantly changing, and that seems perfectly obvious. The cycle of change from night to day, from season to season, and our own cycle of birth, growth, maturing, decay and death. Nothing stays still, yet this constant change can be difficult and painful, but within this change part of us longs for stability and security.

Mary brought her four-month-old baby to the surgery as he had gone off his food and was not sleeping so well at night. She had done very well as a single young mother caring for her child on her own, and it was unusual for her to be concerned. I examined the baby and told her she was quite fit. She said that, in that case, the baby's illness was probably caused by her recent move. She was not happy with her new lodgings, as the tenants smoked and did not seem trustworthy. She realised the baby had sensed she was not at ease and had become unwell. She decided to move again at the first opportunity. Once they were settled again, the baby returned to her former good health.

But it is not only changes like moving house or a new job that can bring on illness; internal changes like changes in belief systems and attitudes can be equally difficult.

Aslam was a successful second-generation Bangladeshi pharmacist with a cheerful, energetic nature who usually kept robust health. So I was surprised to see him in the surgery. He had been experiencing headaches and dizzy spells and was concerned that if he had a serious illness it would affect his business. All his five children had done well at school, so I asked how they were getting on. He sighed, and with an air of resignation recounted how his second daughter had taken up with a non-Moslem, and wanted to marry him. As he described his anguish he began to realise how all this internal turmoil was affecting his health. He did not ask for any investigations or treatment, and departed saying how difficult it was for him with his own traditional beliefs to accept the ways of this modern generation. He knew that, until he could do so, the symptoms would continue.

Children long for and need a stable environment to flourish and they can be very sensitive to any change that they perceive as a threat to their security.

John at ten was brought to the surgery by his parents because in the last six months he had been bedwetting. Not an uncommon problem, but one often caused by family upset. I examined him and did some simple tests which eliminated a physical cause. I asked John how he got on at school and about his home life. Quite unexpectedly he revealed he felt alone, and deserted by his father. Both parents were shocked at this revelation. It transpired that John's father had not been spending much time with his son as pressures at work meant he often came home from work late. At a review visit his mother told me her husband had changed his schedule and now always made a point of getting home in time to read John bedtime stories. Together they had become keen on making model planes and went off flying them at weekends. As a result, John's bedwetting had ceased.

Not all cases of family disharmony adversely affecting the children are as easily resolved as John's. It is so important for children to feel supported throughout periods of change. When parents are separated or constantly rowing children often do not get the attention they need. Parents may not fully realise the damage they are inflicting on their children, not only in the short term but for years to come. Upsets outside the home can equally adversely affect a child.

Shaun was now twelve and I had known him and his family since his birth. His mother said he was having problems with constipation. Shaun had always been a bright, fun-loving youngster, but now he did not look too happy. It only took a few questions to establish that he was being bullied at school. The parents were unaware of what was happening, and were shocked at this revelation. Fortunately it all was resolved quickly, and in a couple of weeks Shaun was back to his usual self. No medication was required, and the constipation got better.

Children at this age are very sensitive and vulnerable, and such bullying is not uncommon and can be quite damaging. Parents need to be alongside their children, and themselves be sensitive to their needs and not put everything down to a bad mood.

Another aspect to consider is that parents can unwittingly contribute to their children's unhappiness by having unrealistic expectations of them. They may wish to mould their children into something rather than help them find their own path. It is rather like a young tree that wants to express its inherent nature freely, but is constantly pruned to meet the idea of how the gardener feels it should look. Many illnesses in adults can be traced back to possibly well-meaning parents restricting their children in finding their own way.

Emma had another flare-up of her eczema, and her mother was concerned that it was keeping her awake at night which interfered with her concentration at school. She was a bright girl in many ways. She was in the top set for most of her subjects, and was particularly gifted in music and art. Her parents supported her in all her activities and knew her eczema often got worse before exams. They were quite open to comple-mentary therapies, and willing to pay if it might help her skin. She was now thirteen, and her mother remarked that she was becoming difficult after being such a compliant child. She commented, 'Emma has a habit of scratching herself when she is told to do anything.'

Somehow I needed to help the parents give Emma more space but it did not seem appropriate to tell her mother that her pushi-ness was to some extent the cause of her daughter's skin complaint. Later her mother consulted with her irritable bowel (caused by her own tension), and when she got help for her problems, Emma's eczema improved.

Adolescence

The change from a child to an adult is difficult for each individual. It can be a tumultuous time for everyone. Besides all the physical changes of puberty, the new emotional feelings, and mentally adapting to external changes such as a new school, there is deeper spiritual change going on. The innocent playful self of childhood is beginning to be overshadowed by the emerging personality. This development of the adult personality is like a cloak that we wrap around us to present to the world. We may not be entirely comfortable with it, and it may alter from time to time, but it is absolutely necessary to cope with the outer world as we develop and grow.

A parent's pleasure should be to see these little souls grow and fly off as free spirits. We should learn from our children, not teach them. The food for their growth is love. Babies require comfort and cuddles. Toddlers fun and games. Youngsters encouragement and support. Adolescents security and listening.

Menopause

The first menstrual period of a girl marks the time when she is changing from childhood to womanhood. The transition is a gradual maturing process over several years, and her first bleeding is a sign of this change. Similarly at the cessation of periods this marks the change from fertile womanhood to the mature woman reaching the autumn of her life. It is an opportunity to look back and assess her achievements, and to look forward towards her future development. At this mid-point in their life other life changes often occur: their own parents may be reaching the end of their lives and their deaths may be the first experience of the death of a close relative. If there are children they may be going through the difficult time of adolescence or leaving home, and there may be the question of finding or changing jobs.

Men do not have the specific symptoms that some women experience, but they too do go through this mid-life crisis. They have similar stressful life changes in the second part of their life. Their life goals at work or in other activities may have been reached, or because of circumstances have failed to be reached and they have to accept that. They may need to set themselves new goals which may involve a new orientation.

The meaning of change

Nothing stays the same, and it is normal and natural that everything goes through a cycle of change. If it seems for the best it is easy to accept, but if not we may ask ourselves why things are altering.

To understand the true meaning of change we do have to approach it in a non-judgemental way. That is, by going with the flow of change, not having expectations, accepting the outcome, and being surprised at how, if we trust things to work out for the best, they invariably do.

The purpose of change in our personal life is to challenge us and encourage us to grow as people. We all are constantly changing our views, our beliefs, our perspectives. What seemed to hold our attention yesterday as important, now has faded. What was a strong belief is no longer so.

Looking back

Much of this book has been devoted to describing ways of releasing the five negative qualities that interfere with our life. Sometimes the wounds run deep and it takes tremendous effort to change and move on. It can be like a physical wound where to achieve optimum healing one has to get right down to the base and clear it out, and only then will the natural healing begin to work.

If you feel a particular person from your past still seems to have a hold on you and you would like to move forward, try this exercise.

Find a quiet time and place. Calm yourself, and still your mind so images can come easily. When you are quite relaxed imagine yourself standing next to the person you want to break free from.

See both of you held together by a strong cord and wherever you go the other person pulls on you. It prevents you moving freely and holds you back. Now take a strong pair of scissors or sharp knife, and as you raise it to cut the cord say to the person that you are now going to cut the link that joins you both. This will allow you both not to depend on each other and have the freedom to go in your own direction. Now, full of purpose, cut the cord. See it break. The other person drifts away, and you are left feeling free. You feel lighter and easier. Surround yourself with an impenetrable golden sphere of light so that you feel safe. Even if you see the person again your sphere of light will prevent them from latching on to you again. They cannot affect you. You are free. Once you have really experienced this in your mind if you do see them again it will be much easier.

Living in the moment

One of the most difficult things to do is to live completely in the moment. Our mind, when not engaged in an immediate task, is either thinking about things that have happened or thinking about the future and so we do not appreciate just where we are as we move through a change. It is like being on a car or train journey: we are thinking about where we are going or have been, and fail to enjoy the travelling itself. When we arrive we may then regret we did not appreciate all that happened on the trip. It is not easy to keep focused in the present completely. Indeed it is a skill that we could all benefit from practising.

Looking forward

Change can be stressful, if we see it as stressful. If you see it as an adventure, it can be a challenge. It can be exciting and fun. As with any problem it is our attitude that is all-important. It is our attitude that determines how we handle change, both the external changes in the world around us, and the internal changes in ourselves. If we can anticipate change and make plans, whatever it is has every chance of going more smoothly. This planning is not just organisational, but to do with planning the attitude to adopt.

Try this when undertaking any task. Think of the positive quality you would like to bring to the task, and what positive quality you would like to achieve at its completion.

Take washing the car. 'I would like to clean it with joy.' Or going for an interview. 'I will be calm and clear. Success is what I expect.' Or starting a new job. 'I will be friendly and make new friends.'

Ritual

Rituals do have a central place in change as they deepen the meaning for the individual and the community. A ritual may look pointless to the outsider, but does give a great depth to the experience of change.

Every society will have their own rituals at death and marriage, and most will have some ritual at birth. They are often part of a religion, and when religion is no longer central to the cultural life, as in most Western countries, these rituals are lost and with them the feeling of occasion. In Europe Celtic societies celebrated the change from each season with festivals of dancing and feasting, and most have been absorbed into the Christian calendar. We will all have our own family rituals of celebrating events such as Christmas, or our own personal rituals of getting up in the morning.

The two main changes that present any problems in a general practice consultation, as I have discussed in this chapter, are the menopause and adolescence. There seems to be no real ritual to mark these changes. Some years ago a group of us met for a day to discuss this problem of lack of ritual. Our conclusion was we should create our own. For example, there could be new dances, or gatherings for celebrations. Some of the ladies of menopausal age in the group met again over a weekend, to share their family life to date. They created poems and songs about letting go of the fertile period of their life. They then turned to making plans for the future.

With my own three daughters when their periods started it meant they could then get their ears pierced. We allowed them to have time off school to go out with their mother and her friends to buy new clothes. They went to their grandmother who gave them a special piece of her own jewellery as a celebration of the change.

With boys there is not such an obvious mark of change at adolescence. For them it may be more of going out to face a challenge. In tribal times it may have been killing a lion, but now could be going off camping on their own for the first time.

The real strength of any ritual is to create it oneself. It is much more than what you do but it has a personal meaningfulness.

Peacefulness

It does seem that the rate of change in the world today has speeded up, so much so that one can feel disorientated and confused. That makes it even more important for each of us to stand back and touch that point of peacefulness within ourselves. Different ways of doing this have already been outlined, but the important thing is to have the intent to set some time aside each day.

Taking this time to stand back and observe where we are is like finding a quiet spot in the middle of a storm. By freezing the moment in the present it gives you a snapshot of where you are now, where you have been, and a view of where you are going. When people consult me as a healer and receive natural healing they often will describe that they feel relaxed and calm, but in addition have a sense of space and stillness. They have a clarity about where they are on their journey, and if they have an illness where the imbalances are, what their illness is telling them, and what they need to do. It is not usually something dramatic, but more often a very practical step, such as needing to cut down hours at work, appreciating their partner more, or doing something with the family.

Peacefulness is not only the goal of optimum healing, it is a very practical way of reaching that goal.

Spiritual Awareness

During the teenage years there is often an opening up at all levels, and this can make individuals of this age more prone to psychic phenomena. This can include telepathy, pre-cognition, spirit communication, and psychokinesis (affecting physical objects with the mind). There are potential negative forces associated with such phenomena and are best not experimented with at a young age. Playing with ouija boards or taking drugs can expose individuals to psychic phenomena and can be quite disturbing. Of course they can be fascinating as they expose us to other dimensions of reality as we perceive it, but are a diversion to the real task of optimum healing.

Soul consciousness

From the moment of conception a life is created, and a beautiful soul is off on its journey. It is our privilege as parents and adults to nurture and love this person. Our job is to give security and encouragement to allow the child to flourish, to be tolerant and understanding. Would it not be a wonderful way to live if we continued to behave that way to adults as well?

As we grow and experience the world it is important to keep a connection to that deeper part of our being. We do need to have a personality, an ego consciousness, to experience the world and all the changes, but the one thing that is constant is our soul.

God consciousness

There does seem to be a more intensive spiritual awareness at the time of the natural transition from child to adult, and from adult to mature elderly. Many people begin to ask spiritual questions, perhaps for the first time. Who am I? What am I doing? Is there a God? These questions can be preoccupying, and can be quite disturbing.

Nicholas heard a talk on the radio about the second coming of Christ, and at the age of fourteen had set off to join a religious sect in London. Fortunately this group were responsible enough to bring him home to his parents. But Nicholas was left disturbed by the experience and felt 'called by God', to bring all sinners to the light. His parents thought he might be suffering from schizophrenia, and brought him to see me for my opinion. After a long discussion I felt we could manage the situation without referral to a psychiatrist. He would, with his parents' support, join the local Baptist youth group, but be encouraged to keep up his school studies. For many years his inner revelation of God drove him in his church work, but he was able to keep to his school work, and play in the football team. After study at college he worked in the church.

This opening up spiritually at that age is very powerful, and can be quite disruptive to everyone involved. For Nicholas, the ground of intellectual work at school and the physical exercises were essential in keeping a balance for his spiritual awakening. It can seem very like a mental illness and needs a lot of understanding by everyone to support the person.

Towards the second half of our life this kind of revelation tends to be less dramatic. It may even seem something that arises out of necessity as the individual begins to question their own mortality. It is perhaps the spiritual task of the second part of our life to address this very question. What is my relationship with God? Not something people will talk much about in private, let alone to their doctor. But I often sense this in patients, especially if they have an illness towards the end of their life.

Collective consciousness

It is the study of nature that can give us the profoundest of insights into our connection to everything. The natural cycle of birth, growth, decay and death is the reality of all things; animal, plants and even planets. We are part of that. It is so simple, yet so mysterious. I am born, I grow, I decay, I die.

'Things are not as they used to be. In the old days it was done better.' How often do we hear that, or say it ourselves? In my experience as a doctor such attitudes make it difficult for patients to accept advice. Perhaps it is the need for security and stability that can cause so much anger and frustration in people when faced with change. This is not only people with analytical minds, but those who view change itself as being abnormal. Behind that is fear of change, and as life is about change they have a fear of life. So simply remind ourselves of how it is; that everything is changing and we must learn to embrace that change. Observe nature and we will learn many useful lessons.

Positive qualities

Remember the child-like qualities
There is a whole list of wonderful qualities that children have that we forget about as we become adults: playfulness, creativity, spontaneousness, openness, inquisitiveness, acceptance, forgiveness, fun-lovingness. We have so much to learn by observing children and becoming more child-like ourselves.

Hold on to your core values
Through all the changes what are the basic values that you feel whatever happens to you will never change? Qualities like honesty, trustworthiness, caringness, that are intrinsically part of you. Honour them and respect them. How can you draw on them to help you through changes?

What qualities would you like?
When you see others managing change well what are the qualities they have? Search out people you know who seem best able to cope with change, and observe what qualities they have. It is often to do with the attitudes they adopt to problems rather than how they organise and manage them. Try to identify their specific qualities, and consider how you can integrate them into your life. Two positive qualities that I think are essential to change are flexibility and lightness.

Flexibility

Flexibility is moving with stillness,
And is going easily.
Flexibility is bending like a reed in the wind
It is having a beginner's mind
Flexibility is going with the flow.

In our own surgery we employ over thirty staff, and several years ago we seemed to lurch from one crisis to the next. The government had introduced radical reforms without any consultation, and we had to adapt very rapidly. No sooner had these reforms been implemented than the rules changed. There were quite serious financial and staffing implications as a result. On top of that, new technology was thrust upon us, several key staff left, and there seemed endless interpersonal staffing problems. Not an unfamiliar story among many professions in recent years. When we took time out to review out position and plan our management for the future we took a key decision. That was to plan to be flexible to be able to cope with what would continue to be a rapid and unpredictable changing situation. Our key value to help us through changing times was flexibility. The practice was split up into small teams that were responsible for their own areas. So as problems arose each was asked to find the solutions themselves rather than ask the management. That included interpersonal disputes. Of course they needed help at first to find ways of facilitating this process. We also made sure that everyone's job could be done by someone else, so that if someone was off sick or left it would not be disruptive. We still have problems, but with an attitude of flexibility they are now seen as challenges rather than stressful.

Lightness

Lightness brightens the way,
And can bring a soft touch.
Lightness overcomes heaviness.
It eliminates darkness.
Light heralds love.

Sometimes when we anticipate change we anticipate a poor outcome. We may have a sense of foreboding that all will not be well. This is fear creeping in. It is good to have due concerns and plan ahead, but not good to harbour irrational fears. This in itself will influence what lies ahead. When this darkness casts a shadow over our thoughts, stop and think of light. Think of a bright beam of light illuminating the scene you have imagined. Flood your thoughts with light. Fill the people with light.

A guide to change

1	Plan for all eventualities.
2	Let go of anything or anyone that holds you back.
3	Withdraw into a moment of peace.
4	Hold to your core values.
5	Remember your child-like qualities.
6	Honour your mature qualities.
7	Be flexible.
8	Live with lightness
9	Death is at the end, but it is not the end. It is another change.

Accidents

∙∙

An old lady tripping over a kerb stone and breaking an ankle, a housewife cutting her finger with a knife, or a child spilling boiling water over himself. Are such accidents a matter of bad luck, misfortune, or simply chance, being in the wrong place at the wrong time? The rational view is that accidents are random events, and there is not much we can do about it.

But perhaps by watching where she was going the old lady could have avoided tripping. If the housewife had not rushed when preparing the food she would not have cut herself, or if the pot was out of reach the child would not have been burned. In other words could they have made some contribution to these accidents?

Accidents and meaning

The healing approach is not one of chance or blame, but that accidents are meaningful events. Everything that happens, including an accident, has a purpose. To take it further we attract what we need, not only to sustain us, but to offer us opportunities to change.

Jack was forty when he crushed his hand so severely he could no longer work as a bank clerk. It seemed at the time a complete disaster. He was forced to retire as he could no longer even count money because of his disability. He had problems with sleeping, and then developed indigestion symptoms which needed some medication. After a year he began to look for another job. He had always wanted to work outside, and applied to work as a postman. The job paid a lot less, but he enjoyed the work, and was much happier. (Incidentally, Jack's indigestion probably meant that he could not digest the fact he had to give up work.) As soon as he had taken the positive step of looking for work once more he no longer required any medication. Years later he told me if it was not for his accident he would still be miserable in his job as a bank clerk.

This opportunity to change may at first not appear obvious, especially if you have been involved in a life-threatening situation. There may be physical injuries to recover from, and often much more difficult emotional upset. One's energy is often taken up in the early stages with the physical recovery, and coming to terms with what has happened. Most people will see as their goal to get back to normal as quickly as possible. *Get over it, forget it, and carry on as before.* To some to reflect on the meaning may seem pointless, and even hinder the recovery process.

An accident at the time may appear a bizarre event, and even if we adopt the healing approach and look for meaning, it can still seem to be the hand of misfortune at work. Yet with the passing of time a new perspective can develop, and the accident offers an opportunity to reflect on our situation and make changes at the right time in our life.

Accidents as challenges

An accident can also challenge the very foundations of our beliefs just at a time when we begin to think that life is well ordered and predictable. An accident is unpredictable, shakes everything up, testing strengths and finding weaknesses. It challenges us to question many of our dearly held views that we live our lives by.

Mrs Sanders, a retired lecturer in mathematics, fell down the stairs injuring her back. The X-rays showed no broken bones, and various therapies over many months only partially helped. She thought it was unjust that she should suffer so much pain, as she felt she had lived a life without blame. For years after her accident she complained bitterly that the medical profession could not help her. Her well-ordered life, with her views of right and wrong, reward and punishment, had been shaken by her accident. She remained bewildered as to why such a chance event could happen to her.

We sometimes build up a wall around us of beliefs and ideas that we think, if we hold to them, will protect us from the harshness of the world. Then one day for some reason the wall breaks, and the world behind the collapsed wall can appear a very different place. We can feel scared, lonely and ill prepared. All we have then is ourselves, as we are forced to fall back on our own inner resources.

Accidents do not challenge only the patient's views and beliefs, but sometimes those of the doctor, as happened to me some years ago.

Mary **Mains was** a medical receptionist from a neighbouring medical practice and had been involved in a car accident. She had been waiting at a train crossing, and a car shunted her from behind. At the time it did not seem very serious. Two weeks later she consulted, complaining of a stiff neck. Examining her, she had reasonable movement of her neck, and I arranged a neck X-ray. This proved normal, so I prescribed some painkillers and hoped the discomfort would resolve in time. It didn't. She was back after a month no better, and still not fit to work. After this visit I referred her for some physiotherapy, and after ten sessions she felt well enough to work again. However after two weeks back at work the pains had returned and she had to stop. It was now six months from the original accident, and neither of us knew what to do next. There were no insurance claims, and she was keen to get back to work. This case had challenged my usual management of whiplash injuries to the neck, so I suggested she could try some healing. After several sessions the pain improved enough for her to return to work, and after two months she was pain-free. I asked the healer what he had done to get her better so quickly. He explained that during the accident Mary's subtle energy field surrounding her body had been knocked out of line, and that had to be put back before the physical body could be corrected. Mary's accident had challenged me to consider a broader view of the human organism. The healer suggested that the human body is more than flesh, bones, blood and organs, but is permeated and surrounded by energy fields which can be disrupted by accidents. This certainly challenges the traditional medical view, and set me off on a study of the subtle energy fields of the human body.

Meaning of disasters

One may ask what can be the possible meaning of disasters such as plane crashes, hurricanes, or earthquakes. What is the positive outcome of them, and what was the personal responsibility of those who suffered or died through them? Not an easy question to answer, especially for those who may have been involved themselves, or lost a loved one. Yet looking for a meaning can be helpful to the survivors. They can attend enquiries, and press for changes in any of the identifiable causal factors.

It seems that the meaning is not so much in the individual area of responsibility, but more at a society level. In an earthquake the houses may have been sited wrongly, or be of inferior construction. Leaders of society involved in the house construction may have been influenced by money, greed and power, rather than by what is best for the people they represent. As members of that society we in turn perhaps do not get involved enough to voice our concerns and influence the leaders. As with personal accidents, disasters shake everything up, lead to questions, challenge us to change.

Mark and his girlfriend were among the survivors of the car ferry disaster, the *Herald of Free Enterprise*, in the English Channel in 1987. Mark had always been a friendly, outgoing person, but for months following the accident he was moody and anti-social. He felt fate had been unkind to him, and he felt powerless and helpless. It was three months before he could face work again, and his relationship with his girlfriend ended.

It took him seven months before he accepted he needed to talk through his experience with a trained counsellor. I can remember two years after he told me that being in the ferry disaster had changed his life in many ways but mainly positively. He had learned so much about himself through the counselling. He had led such a sheltered life before, and only really considered himself. The accident had made him feel fortunate and have a greater compassion for others. It also produced positive action by governments. As you may know, the regulations concerning the construction of ferries, and safety procedures were improved following an enquiry.

With disasters or serious accidents it is not uncommon to have 'flashbacks' of the accident so the whole terror of the situation is relived with the same intensity of feeling. It is now over fifty years since the end of the Second World War, and I still have wives who tell me their husbands wake up screaming about events they had witnessed during the war. Most men of that generation had seen some atrocities, and suffered the horrors of war. The culture at the time was to keep it to oneself, many suffered, and go on suffering still. Sharing the story even years later is helpful. As it is retold it loses some of the fear. Another technique that one can use on one's own is to see the incident played on a television screen and turn down the volume and fade the colour. Imagining standing back from the screen, and viewing it further back makes the whole thing less intense.

Destiny

Is the course of our life predetermined even before we are born, or is the opposite true, that we are totally responsible for everything we do? The first approach, which is fatalistic, tends to rob us of our power and freedom, while the latter can leave us the burden of guilt.

The healing answer to the question of destiny is both these answers and neither. It does seem we are born with a life plan, like a route map to a destination. The goal is the same for everyone, and that is to find the peacefulness of enlightenment. The route that we take is predetermined to the extent that we are born to certain parents, in a particular country, at a particular time in history. In addition we have our physical attributes and innate skills. Within that restriction we do have the freedom to do what we like. Destiny may be hidden through layers of family and cultural processing. The next case shows that we do have the power to change even that destiny.

James came from an Eastern Jewish background. He showed me a lump on the side of his face which looked like a growth, and I said I needed to refer to a specialist. He told me he expected it would be cancer as most of his family had died of cancer. Only recently his younger sister had just been diagnosed as having breast cancer.

Two weeks later the surgeon confirmed that he did have a malignant growth. It would require surgical removal. James was a man who had practised meditation since his early twenties, and knew the power of the mind. He thought if the body could make new tissue perhaps it could also dissolve the tumour. He began to sense that it was his destiny to cure this cancer, and so break the family taboo of cancer. He went for a silent intense meditation retreat of four weeks, and gradually the cancer in his jaw shrank and disappeared. The extraordinary thing was that when he contacted his sister her breast lump had begun to regress. Her own doctor was astonished when after four months her malignant lump had gone.

At a deeper level we each have something to fulfil in this lifetime. Finding what that is, and trying to follow it, is our individual and unique task. When we are on the right path we feel full of energy, and may even experience an enthusiastic certainty. It is when we wander too far off the path that we become unhappy, lose the sense of purpose, feel tired, and are not content. Outwardly our life may be very difficult physically, emotionally and mentally, but it is the spiritual strength of knowing what we are doing to be right that sustains us through the difficult times.

So destiny is not like fate. With destiny, there is a route plan for each of us that we first have to discover, then do our best to follow. It means that every event, including accidents, is part of our destiny.

Unusual experiences

Accidents can provide opportunities to glimpse other aspects of reality which are beyond our perception of everyday living. At first patients can seem reluctant to share their experiences. If they feel someone will listen sympathetically it is a relief to tell someone who thinks they are not going out of their mind, have had some kind of brain injury, or are making it up. These are real experiences and are far commoner than one might think.

One observation is that time seems to slow down. Everything appears much clearer, and things can happen in slow motion. I experienced this slowing down of time myself once when I fell twenty feet off a ladder. I was cutting a branch off a tree with a chainsaw when I slipped. From that point it was as if time had almost stopped, and I was able to consider what was the best thing to do. I can clearly recall thinking that I had to throw the saw away from me, and remember to break my fall by landing like a parachutist. I did that and to my surprise I got up uninjured.

Another experience people recall during a life-threatening accident is that all the events of their life are played out in front of them. It seems to take an age, but in reality could only be a few seconds.

Sheila was involved in a car accident, and had experienced one of these moments of clarity. She had not sustained any injuries, but the accident had upset her considerably. Through tears she described that a car coming towards her lost control, and hit the car she was travelling in side on. She said, 'Just before the impact everything came to the fore.' 'Everything' was her boyfriend's death two years before. She was about to leave home before his death, but now at the age of thirty-three she still lived with her parents. The accident had brought all the conflicting feelings and thoughts into her mind with an intensity in that moment that held her attention. She went to see a bereavement counsellor, and as a result revealed that she had been sexually abused as a child. Slowly over the months she talked through these issues, and eventually left home to live in another town.

Extraordinary things happen in accidents that not everyone is willing to talk about. Some people report that they have felt the presence of a beneficial being intervene at a critical moment. My own son fell fifteen feet off our garage roof head-first on to a concrete forecourt. When he told me I was surprised he had only had a knee graze. It was later that he said as he was falling he felt a large hand hold him, and turn him so that he landed feet first.

I have heard other people describe similar happenings that they attribute to their guardian angel.

George Atkin appeared in the surgery with his leg in plaster. He had always been a keen climber, and told me how he happened to be in a plaster. He was climbing on a mountain in Scotland, and had broken his ankle after a fall. He lay for several hours in the snow, separated from his backpack which contained all his emergency kit. The situation seemed hopeless, and he was resigned to dying where he was. From nowhere a man appeared out of the mist, helped bandage his leg, get into warm clothes out of his rucksack, and gave him a warm drink. He then disappeared into the mist. Not only was that an unusual event, but the leader of the rescue party said the moment George was reported missing the name of the crag where he was stranded came into his head. They made straight for the place, and when they found him the following day they could not believe what good condition he was in. The man who had helped George was never traced, and how the rescue party found him was described as a chance in a thousand. This experience had a profound effect on George, and he resolved to do something worthwhile with his life, and began by working for a local charity.

Peacefulness and accidents

Sometimes people involved in accidents experience a deep sense of peace in the middle of the most extreme situation. This is almost the complete opposite to what one would expect. It could be the first time in their life they have experienced such a profound peacefulness.

Madeline told me about such an experience she had just at the point she feared that she would certainly die, when she crashed her car over a bridge. She felt this deep sense of peace. She described the peace as beyond description and it filled and surrounded her. It took her many months to recover from her physical injuries and psychological trauma. She said that, undoubtedly, the experience of peace gave her the strength to endure the many operations and discomfort she suffered.

Experiences at life-threatening accidents are often similar to near-death experiences. People describe moving away from their body, and going towards a comforting light. There may be friends or relatives present, and they have a feeling of great peacefulness. These experiences are not only intense, but quite personal. They have a mystical quality to them, and a mere description fails to convey the effect it has had on the individual. As a result they often seem to develop the spiritual quality of tolerance towards themselves and others.

One word of warning about some of these intense spiritual experiences is that they can cause a spiritual arrogance. The person thinks that the revelation they have experienced is a unique experience, and that they have been specially chosen. They think they have some special status and a mission to tell others about their experience. However the truly spiritual person demonstrates their spirituality through their actions in a quiet way.

The above stories demonstrate important experiences under dramatic conditions but one does not have to wait for an accident to experience such peacefulness. It can be done by using the natural capacity of our minds to think in pictures, and using the mind to concentrate on particular calming and pure images.

The white sphere

Find a quiet place, sit comfortably, and breathe naturally. Imagine a sphere, about the size of your head; see it above your head as a radiant white ball. Concentrate on that image for several minutes, and as other images and thoughts appear send them away so you always return to the pure white sphere. This sphere of light has a great relaxing effect, and sends out beams of calm. As you look at it, you begin to feel its effect. It gradually decreases in size, not losing any of its potency, until it is about one centimetre across. It descends through the top of your head to find its place in the centre of your chest. Then that profound peacefulness begins to expand to fill every organ in your body, to circulate in your blood vessels, to infuse your bones, and reach every cell. It is warm, relaxing, and helps you feel totally at ease with yourself and the world. It begins to affect the area around your body, and fill the whole room. Try to hold the image and the feelings for as long as you can without any distraction. This may only be for a few seconds, but after some practice you may be able to capture the experience for several minutes.

Spiritual awareness and accidents

Soul consciousness

With some life-threatening accidents some people report out-of-body experiences. They feel separate from their body, emotions and even thinking. They have the impression of witnessing what is happening to them. It is really the same as the 'near-death experience', and whether they are literally out of their body looking down has never really been proven one way or the other. However it gives us some idea of experiencing soul consciousness without the distraction of a body and mind.

ric had tripped while walking on a cliff path and had fallen thirty feet on to a ledge below. Later he was to learn he had broken both his legs, fractured his skull, and torn some internal organs. As he lay there he said he experienced himself outside his body, and had a certainty that it was a soul. He could see this person, whom he recognised was himself, lying on the cliff edge below him in a curious detached way. Not only did he not have any pain, but was quite neutral in his emotions. He was interested in what his rescuers were doing, and was not concerned what happened to himself. The next thing he remembers is waking up in a hospital bed in a lot of pain.

In recent years there has been quite a lot of research to try to prove that these experiences are real, and that people really are outside their body and not just imagining it. It is not an easy subject to research, and to date there are only a few convincing cases where people who were unconscious can describe details of their accident that could only have been known if they had been watching. No matter, such experiences can have a profound effect. Some see it as a deep insight into their true self, and that gives them a new perspective on life. Others with the same experience will disregard it. It may be because they cannot accept it as real, and continue to live their life as before. The experience is often just too much for them to take in.

God consciousness

It is interesting that very few people with unusual experiences in accidents, in near-death experiences, and in other altered states such as dreams rarely report having met God. There are few reports of God as a father or mother figure, or as any of the other representations we might commonly see or read about. What people do report is a sense of a beneficial and comforting presence, which is so profound yet simple it is difficult to describe. Is that experience God? Who knows?

John, now in his fifties, works as a truck driver. He was brought up a Protestant, and after studying Catholicism abandoned it to become a confirmed non-believer. One winter's evening he was involved in one of those dreadful pile-up crashes in the fog on the motorway, and felt sure at the time he was going to die. Immediately after the moment of impact he felt a presence which he could only describe as love which totally surrounded and filled him. He knew this presence to be God. It took six months to recover from the accident, but the experience transformed his life. He now has a certainty of God through direct experience. He did not join any religious group, and carried on in his job as a truck driver. He said people often commented to him how he now looked different, as though he had an inner glow, and that is how he said he felt. John's spiritual belief was simple. Simply, to him, God is love.

Collective consciousness

Once more sometimes an accident can give an insight into this experience.

Dennis had fallen and could not get up because of a twisted ankle after tumbling while skiing. The problem was he had gone off the main track and where he had fallen was out of sight and earshot of anyone. As he lay there he realised that unless he was rescued he would freeze overnight in the snow. After several hours he began to drift in and out of consciousness, and after his recovery he had one clear memory of that time. He had an image of a rose. There it was with a striking clarity, beauty and perfection. He wondered at the thought, that all roses were equally perfect, and beautiful in their own way. He thought that is how every human being is. The image only lasted a few seconds. But it was a very intense experience. He could remember it now with the same clarity, although it was eighteen years ago. It filled him with a sense of joy, and helped him to see the beauty in everything and everyone. Like many such experiences they are very personal, and are difficult to convey in words. But he told me that experience did give him some insight into the idea that each person is a soul, and every soul contains the same beautiful qualities, and in that way we are all linked.

Spiritual qualities and accidents

Trust

Trust is an essential quality for optimum healing: that all will be well and that all my needs will be met.

Trust means more than belief and is even more than faith. It is a deep knowing that what will be is meant to happen. Every single event in life has a purpose, and this includes the unpredictable and, sometimes, disasters. It sounds easy to have trust, but how does one gain such a positive attitude, and be able to live a life of total trust?

Like most healing practices it is quite simple, but one needs to try. I discovered this by thinking that when I needed a car space outside a shop I would imagine a free parking space would magically appear. When it did I was at first surprised and a bit taken aback. I found the more I trusted this would happen, the more likely I was to find an empty space. Now apply this to other aspects of your life where you trust that other things will work out for the best. Not that you will get what you want, but what you need. By having trust your life can change. It is with this trust you can see that your real life's purpose begins to unfold. You begin to trust it will; and it does.

Trust is knowing that everything has a purpose,
And all will be well.
It is being responsible,
And letting go of responsibilities
Trust is knowing that we have done our best.

Some people do seem to be accident-prone and they are the sort who tend to say, 'I am always unlucky. Things never work out for me. Everything ends up badly.'

Remember action does follow thought and, to reverse your luck, begin to think in a positive way. Begin by saying such affirmations as 'I am lucky. Today I will have good fortune. Things will turn out for the best. I trust all will be well.' Then they will.

Accident prevention

1 Be aware
Pay attention to your attitudes and feelings. In South Africa the workers in the gold mines have a superstition that if they trip over the doormat on the way to work they don't go. But perhaps it is telling them that they are not completely paying attention on that day, which could be fatal in such a dangerous job.

2 Check your intuition
Check inwardly that any situation is right for you. This is not necessarily an easy thing to do, but with practice your intuition will

become finely tuned. It will not always be right, but is a good counter-balance to the rational decision-making process.

3 Observe yourself

Are you physically fit enough for the task? Fathers race at school sports day is the one that always produces a good crop of accidents, as fathers try to prove to themselves that they can still do the hundred yards in the same time as they did in their school days.

Are you emotionally calm? Some women tend to avoid making important decisions just before menstruation as they feel out of sorts during that time of the month. Of course men have their time of the month too for emotional imbalance!

Are you mentally relaxed? If you are worried and on edge whatever you do will be prone to accident.

Are you spiritually of the right attitude? Check if you are wanting to achieve your goal through pride, greed, or ambition.

4 Be prepared

Preparing for any task lessens the risk of accidents. That is not only true of physical and organisational problems, but for mental and emotional tasks as well. The best way to prepare spiritually is to imagine the best outcome, or choose a quality that would help you achieve it.

5 Avoid excess risk

It is good to take some risk, and that is the time we often gain new learning experiences. But only take a risk if you feel ready to. It is common sense not to do so when you are tired, have drunk alcohol or are taking medication.

Advice following an accident

1   **Rest.** Wanting to rest after the shock of an accident is quite natural. Children, even after a minor accident, often sleep for hours. After a serious accident resting does not only give you a chance to recover physically, but time to assess how it has affected you. However, feeling progressively drowsy after

a head injury can be an indication of serious cerebral bleeding and medical advice should be sought.

2   **Share your experience.** This consists of two parts. First tell someone in detail what happened factually, and second how you feel about the whole experience. This type of debriefing is essential soon afterwards, and needs to be repeated later. The person who shares your story needs to be a good listener, and may need to be a trained counsellor.

3   **Get medical advice.** Muscular strains following accidents which initially can appear quite minor have a way of becoming chronic if not attended to early. Physiotherapy, osteopathic and chiropractic manipulation early on can prevent problems developing later.

4   **Hold no grudges.** However much you feel it was the other person's fault, remember negative emotions, if held on to, will affect you.

5   **Be wary of court cases.** It is well recognised throughout the medical profession that where there is a court claim for compensation, the symptoms rarely get better until the claim is settled. That can sometimes take years.

6   **Search for a meaning.** Why did the accident happen now, and in what way has it changed my life? The difficult question to ask of oneself is, 'In what way was I responsible for the accident?'

7   **Look for positive outcomes.** Despite the trauma and injuries an accident can bring out the best in people, bring families and communities together, and highlight problems that need to be resolved.

8   **Trust.** Adopt a positive trusting outlook.

Old Age

Grey hair, a drooping stature and wrinkled skin; muddled and confused. Is that your idea of an old person? Such a description is certainly not true of many older people I know. Some are still playing tennis in their seventies; swimming in their eighties; and managing on their own at home in their nineties. Often old people have a zest for life that is lacking in those much younger. Energy and optimism are certainly aspects of optimum healing and it is possible to have these qualities when elderly.

Old people are frequently labelled by society as being past their 'sell-by date'. They are no longer seen as useful, are helpless, and are a drain on resources. No wonder that so many older people have a negative attitude about their age. Typical comments I hear every day are: 'It is not much fun getting old.' 'Old age is downhill all the way.' 'I can no longer enjoy the things I used to.' 'Nothing can be done because of my age.' 'I am too old to change my ways.'

A lady with a different attitude was Bertha Johnson. At eighty-four her recent problem was pain in her chest. As her doctor I knew that there were many possible causes of her discomfort. Heart disease, arthritis, infection and malignancy all had to be considered. I examined her and thought her pain was most likely to be due to muscular strain. She remembered what happened. Two weeks before she had been dancing in her kitchen to pop music and got carried away with the rhythm, had slipped and twisted her side. She then went on to explain that she had always enjoyed dancing, and was not going to give it up just because of her age. When she was leaving she said with a twinkle in her eye that she must be more careful next time. She certainly did not think age should stop her doing the things that she wanted to.

The body in old age

The age at which our body is at its peak really depends on what we want to use it for. If we want the flexibility of a gymnast, between ten and eighteen seems to be the best age. For energy and strength in contact sports such as football and rugby, the optimum age is twenty to thirty. Other physical activities that require skill, stamina and endurance may reach their peak up to the mid-forties.

The media has an influence in persuading us what is the acceptable physical look. That almost without exception is a youthful body. The implication is that anything that is not young is undesirable. Grey hair implies worn out and decaying rather than a sign of authority and respect. Wrinkles may mean deteriorating attributes, and not an indication of experience. These distorted opinions of how it is desirable to look for ever youthful is something as individuals we do not have to accept. Because that is all they are: someone's opinion. It is not the truth.

There is a need to take a more positive attitude to older people, and to ourselves when we are older. Not to see the body deteriorating, but to view it as vital and healthy will give it more of an opportunity to be so and it is more likely to be so. It needs looking after with a good diet and regular exercise in the same manner as it would when younger. At the same time we have to listen to what it is saying, and accept our limitations. It is a matter of getting the right balance.

Mental aspects of old age

It is said that after we reach twenty the brain stops growing, and we begin to lose brain cells. From then on we begin to deteriorate and grow old. On the other hand the brain has huge reserves of capabilities which we never use. Most people remain as mentally sharp in their sixties as they were in their twenties. Perhaps only in their eighties do they begin to slow up gradually in some tasks. Short-term memory and calculations may start to decline.

One old lady I know with a deteriorating memory retains a very positive attitude to her problem. When trying to remember something she does not say she cannot remember but, 'I know that, but just give me a bit longer to remember.'

Older people are not so good at dealing with unfamiliar situations. However, such shortcomings are usually adequately compensated for by their experience. A good example is driving a motor car. An old person can be quite proficient on roads they know well, but if faced with a new situation they can be quite disorientated. Fortunately most elderly drivers appreciate their limitations, and will restrict themselves to driving on familiar roads. This use of past skills allows many ninety-year-olds to manage quite reasonably in their own homes with only the minimum of outside support.

Spiritual aspects of old age

It is sad to see people who are so focused on their bodies that they will spend a lot of money attempting to stop the natural ageing process. Patients visit plastic surgeons to have wrinkles removed, and other parts of their body reshaped in an attempt to try to recapture their youth. But we are not just bodies. It is the inner self that is important.

However, there are common fears in old age that have to be faced to find optimum healing. The four main fears of old age are: death, disability, dementia, loneliness.

Death

Death is perhaps the single most unspoken fear in Western society, and is discussed in some detail in the next chapter. Save to say now, as one gets older the reality of death comes closer.

Disability

It is true that the chances of the disabilities of blindness, deafness, paralysis and incontinence are more likely as one gets older.

Worrying about whether it can happen to you is unhelpful. However if you have got some disability, the optimum healing approach is to be accepting, and look positively towards the future. After all, many people are disabled from birth and have had happy and productive lives.

The fear of disabilities is one thing, but many elderly people have a fear of being a burden on others. They do not want to disrupt the lives of their own children and have them look after them. However their children and relatives may want the opportunity to care for them and so pay back the love they received.

Doris, who was now in her nineties, was unable to feed herself, and was incontinent following a stroke. She said that it was ironic that a helpless baby who makes constant demands with feeding and changing is lavished with care and affection, but the elderly who have already contributed so much are often only grudgingly helped by a few.

Giving and receiving is a positive exchange, and just as a mother gets pleasure from caring for her child, a carer gets pleasure from giving love and attention to the old and disabled.

Dementia

As one gets older there is a natural decline in some mental abilities. Although the long-term memory can usually be quite clear, shorter-term memory is not so good. Sometimes the mental functions deteriorate much more rapidly than one would expect for the person's age, and this is known as senile dementia, or Alzheimer's Disease. Again, short-term memory loss is an early first sign, to be followed by difficulty with intellectual tasks such as counting money. In the early stages there can be confusion and anxiety. A depression can develop because the patient still has some insight into the fact that the mental abilities are deteriorating. I have seen some cases of dementia in people in their forties and early fifties who cannot even remember their own name or recognise their husband or wife. This can be very distressing for them as they realise what is happening early on, and can be very difficult for the family.

Although one may no longer be able to communicate with the sufferer in the usual way contact can be kept by others means. The words used are not as important as the way the words are said. See them as the person you love, and communicate with patience and affection. Touch is very important. So holding hands, or massaging feet or shoulders makes a physical connection that goes much deeper. Music, particularly old songs that they may have known when younger, can stimulate the memory. What is important is that they are still the same unique soul despite their deteriorating mental abilities. We can connect through our hearts, which is the link of compassion. Even the severely demented can pick that up. It is our state of being that is critical, whether carer, or professional helper, that determines the quality of communication.

Loneliness

Loneliness is perhaps the biggest problem of the elderly in modern society. Loneliness is the fear of being deserted, and being all alone. There can be plenty of people around, but loneliness is that unpleasant feeling of being apart. It is the loss of intimacy and being able to share your life with others. Not only the problems, but the little things. The pleasures of sharing a joke, commenting on a news item, or of ordering something for the house. Life outwardly goes on as before, but inwardly can seem boring and pointless. It is most acutely felt after the death of a loved one, and is the most lasting of all the feelings of grief.

Mrs Watkins lived in a lovely bungalow by the sea. She was financially well off, but readily admitted she was unhappy because of her loneliness. Her husband had been dead for fifteen years, and she had no family or friends. She had always been a loner, and thought it was now her fate to have no one to share a conversation with. There were plenty of luncheon clubs and societies for the elderly in the village, but she felt she would never get on with others as people didn't like her. She asked for pills to make her feel better. The end of her life seemed to her to be heading to its futile conclusion.

If you are lonely you need to put such reservations to one side, and simply ask for help. There are many professional and voluntary organisations willing to help, not only in practical ways, but as a befriending service. People really do want to help, and do want the opportunity to be of some service.

A **popular figure at** the golf club, George, a retired diplomat, enjoyed the first ten years of his retirement. He then had a stroke which prevented him playing golf, but he was able to do a bit around the house. His wife had come to consult me as she was concerned because most of the day he sat in front of the television. He told her he felt incompetent, socially inept, and now unlovable. He missed his friends and their companionship. This loss of his social life was a shattering blow to him. I suggested to his wife to contact some of his old friends and invite them to visit. It so happened that one of them had also had a stroke and together they joined the local stroke club and made new friends.

Make friends now. The world is full of interesting people, each with their own stories and particular gifts. Open your heart and approach them. Listen to their lives and share yours. Be friends with as many people as possible. Practise every time you meet someone new. Treat them as you would want them to treat you. Do not be judgemental, and be generous.

Preventing loneliness means going out and making new contacts with young and old alike. Extend your social contacts. With advancing years one needs to cultivate new friendships, and not just rely on established friends. If you retire at sixty-five you could easily live for another fifteen to twenty years, plenty of time to forge good friendships.

FRIENDSHIP: REFRESHES THE SOUL AND BANISHES LONELINESS

What are the qualities you would look for in a friend? Put another way, what qualities can you offer in a friendship? Here are some suggestions from various patients I asked who were lonely.

A friend:

- is a sounding board for half-formed thoughts and ideas;
- offers comfort, reassurance and support;

- listens, and gives positive advice;
- leaves you feeling better;
- knows what you need without asking;
- is for sharing with, not only our grief and problems, but laughter and joy.

The meaning of getting old

Finding a purpose is an important dimension of optimum healing in all ages, but the elderly do have the time and experience for discovering a special role for themselves.

John came to the surgery because he was putting on weight since his wife died two years before. When I asked him what he did with his time, he said he sat and watched television all day, and mostly he found that boring. He ate snacks in front of the TV as he could not be bothered to cook. He had felt useful looking after his wife after her stroke, but now she was gone life seemed empty. He was absorbed in his own misery, and rejected any help. Following this visit I asked the district nurse to weigh him, and advise on his diet. This led to her encouraging him to help out at a disabled club she ran. Her enthusiasm rubbed off on him, and he ended up running the club himself.

Retirement as a word creates the wrong attitude. It suggests one can now retire from life. Having worked hard all your life you are entitled to take it easy for a while, but it should be seen as an opportunity to develop oneself, to use your experience and be of service to others.

If only old people realised how much they have to offer to others. Time, experience and a willingness to be involved are all invaluable qualities they have. In return it will give them a sense of purpose to their life.

It may be unfashionable in this modern age to offer our service free of charge. But voluntary work, where we give ourselves freely, is one of the most rewarding activities to be involved in. Even a few hours a week will be worthwhile. In my small community there are many remarkable old people who can be an inspiration to us all.

For example, our local railway station was overgrown by weeds until two old ladies who used the station regularly were indignant at the mess. They pestered the station manager to give them the tools to tidy up the station, and got the help of a youth group. All the plants were paid for by local companies, and they plan to go on improving the garden for some years yet.

I also have a patient who took up running at sixty, and has run four marathons. A lady of sixty-two who learned to swim after a hip replacement, and a retired accountant in his eighties who acts as a helper on a sailing ship for disabled people.

Finding meaning by reminiscing

Looking back on the good times helps you feel better in the present. Thoughts are focused on happy events, and what you think is what you feel. So it is beneficial to reminisce. A fun birthday party, a happy holiday or place you have been to, and people you have met. How someone helped you through difficult times, a friendly gesture, a smile. These are all things in our treasure-store of memories. Share them with others to cheer them up. It can also give a sense of completion and satisfaction as we approach the end of our life. Offloading some held-back bad memory also helps the healing.

Mrs Corby was a physically and mentally fit seventy-year-old who only occasionally visited the surgery. Her second husband had died three years previously, and she seemed to have coped well with the bereavement. During one of her visits she began to talk about herself, and tell her life story. She had been brought up in the country in a large family, and her main memory was one of hard work and feeling hungry. Her house had been bombed in the war, and she had been homeless for some years. Later on she divorced after learning that her husband had had a mistress for some years. Her only daughter died at the age of thirty-eight, and now she had no surviving relatives. This was a tale of great tragedy, and also one of courage. Throughout her many difficulties she had always tried to be honest, cheerful and caring for others. These were the values that had sustained her through her life. As she was leaving she said she had never told this to anyone before. She felt it was a relief to share her feelings, and I was honoured that she had done so.

Spiritual awareness

As a generalisation the first half of life is about establishing our personality, and reaching goals such as getting a job, buying a home, having a family and fulfilling ambitions. The second half of life is more concerned with finding ourselves, and preparing for death. The first is about outer goals, the second an inner journey of optimum healing.

As we get older, and reflect on our life, we realise that perhaps we have set only the outer goals: financial security, a house, success for our children. If these are met that is good, but if not has life been a failure?

Soul consciousness

Usually as a person gets older there are fewer responsibilities towards others. Your children may have grown up and left home, and the pressures of work should have eased. This means there will be more time for yourself, to get to know yourself better. More time to explore who you truly are. That person inside, who perhaps has been neglected because of busy-ness over the years.

Now is the opportunity to reflect on this most central of life questions. Who am I? Am I more than just this body and mind? If so what am I like stripped of an outer identity of body and personality?

All that has gone before has been in preparation to answer this question of 'Who am I?' The hardships, the problems, the challenges and the moments of joy have all been part of your life to help forge an answer. A unique answer.

Collective consciousness

The time that becomes available as you get older is a marvellous opportunity to deepen that sense of oneness that sometimes we experience in nature. Watching a bird build its nest. Caring for a plant. Going for walks in a forest or along a seashore can give a glimpse of the wider meaning to life. Perhaps for the first time we can reflect on the great abundance of beauty that is all around us. We can breathe in its essence, inhale the vibrancy, absorb the sheer joy. This is what gives us the energy to keep the spirit young.

This inward-looking contemplative approach is not a retreat into introspective emptiness that some people might imagine. On the contrary, it adds to our life experience.

God consciousness

Finally, as you begin to experience a deeper part of yourself and that connection to everything around, you may begin to get a sense of something other. A greater being whom you can communicate with, and who cares for you. This supreme being is the one aspect of life you can totally rely on.

Peacefulness

In old age many tasks in life have been completed. Families brought up, ambitions realised, and perhaps things achieved, so there is plenty of time to devote to discover that inner peacefulness which is at the centre of all human consciousness. This is not an empty time, but one where this search for inner peace is a deepening and enriching experience.

Spiritual qualities. What keeps you young?

As described in the first section of this book optimum healing is enhanced by releasing the negative and improving our positive qualities. These qualities act like an inner glow which spreads their light and warmth to all levels of our being. The two qualities that help to keep you young in spirit are optimism and wisdom, but first a story about an elderly patient called Lily who chose her own three qualities to help to come to terms with her own disabilities due to arthritis.

L **ily was visiting** a bed-bound lady ten years her senior who was blind. The blind lady told her that her approach to her life consisted of the 'three As': accept, adjust, achieve. This made my patient with the arthritis appreciate how fortunate she was in comparison. She was so full of admiration for the courage her blind friend showed that she too decided to adopt the 'three As' as a motto in her life.

Besides this spiritual approach, taking account of physical and mental limitations, forward planning is helpful for disabled patients. Simple modifications in the house can reduce hazards. Improving lighting, and having extra hand rails to get in and out of the bath, or off the toilet. Placing electrical switches up from ground level, hand rails by stairs. Higher chairs can make it easier to get off a seat, and walking frames make the difference in getting around. Consider using different tools for the garden so you can still look after it. Finally, if you have to stop driving your car it is not the end of the world. Very often ordering a taxi can be cheaper than paying for the running and upkeep of a car. If you can, try cycling or walking.

Optimism

Man has searched for the elixir of youth over the years and centuries in order to regain that youthful zest. However it is not to be found in old magic potions, modern medicines, or genetically engineered hormones. We all possess it, and have the ability to develop it. The magic ingredient that keeps us young is having an attitude of optimism.

Optimism is looking forward with hope,
And is daring to live dangerously.
Optimism is retaining a sense of adventure.
It is having a zest for life.
Optimism is looking on the bright side of life.

You are only as old as you think. If you think about it there are those in their twenties who have the characteristics we often attribute to the older generation. Boring, tire easily, no interests, and contribute little to society. It is an optimistic attitude that gives one the ability to find joy and happiness.

One may well ask how can you become optimistic when things do not look too good in the present, and the future does not look too bright either. You may not have too much money, friends may have died, and you may be limited by your disabilities. What you do have control over is your own mind and the attitude you take. Mr Spencer is a good example and he embodies three helpful tips.

Having just returned from a holiday in the Canadian Rockies, Mr Spencer asked if he was fit to go to China. He was now eighty-four years old and three years before had had a major operation for bowel cancer with a colostomy. His wife had died two years previously, and he had no dependants. Furthermore he was limited in his walking because of arthritis, and his sight and hearing were not so good. He had read up on Chinese history, and was keen to walk along the Great Wall of China. How could one say no to a man of such vitality? He was going to live every moment left to him as fully as possible, in a generous and enthusiastic way.

1   Imagine the best outcome

If you are thinking about the future, perhaps planning a holiday, or even just going to a friend's do not think of the problems that could occur. Imagine the best possible outcome. See how you would like things to happen, and consider every detail. For example, if you are going shopping, imagine you find all the things you want to buy are in the shops, and not only that they are of excellent quality. Try to see them, their colour, texture and smell. Imagine you meet a friend and have a chat. You are invited out. You hear some good news. The weather is perfect, and you are offered a lift home. Even if you do foresee difficulties think of ways of overcoming them, rather than dwelling on something that has not yet happened. In this way you create a positive attitude for yourself, and although everything that you wished to happen may not, at least you are improving the chances by thinking about it.

2 Take risks

Start something new. Develop a new interest. Try golf, bridge, or dancing. Go to a class, study a new subject, or learn a new skill. What does it matter what other people may say or think? They may think you foolish. So what, at least you are out to enjoy yourself.

Do not be influenced by others. Very often family and friends out of fear will influence you towards caution. Doctors and social workers are not exempt from taking quite a pessimistic view of the future. You have not got that much time left, so make the most of it. Do what you always wanted to do. It is so important at all ages to create opportunities to have fun. Go out to the theatre and dress up. Have a party. Having an optimistic view, being positive, gives a feeling of liveliness.

3 Let go

When you are older you usually have fewer responsibilities. Your children will have grown up and probably left home. You have done your bit in educating and looking after them, and you must allow them to go their own way. It is a waste of energy worrying about them now. Of course you will retain a real concern about their welfare, but it is a matter now of letting go. Your priority is to yourself, spending the remainder of your days developing your own qualities.

Coping with ageing is a balance between accepting what you are no longer able to do, and keeping that independent zest for life.

Wisdom

Wisdom is knowing we are all the same,
And yet are uniquely different.
Wisdom is learning from experience.
It is drawing on our inner resources.
Wisdom is the King of all qualities.

Wisdom is a quality that matures with age. But it is not just simply having experience through a long life that endows one with some wisdom, but learning from the experiences. For example when we are angry, if we can identify what made us angry we may have added a little to our store of wisdom. On the other hand if at the age of ninety-eight we still talk with anger, we have gained little from the long years.

Wisdom is the courage to go on learning. Learning to let go of the need to please others, and to love without looking for any return. There is a shift of values from wanting to giving, with the emphasis on caring. This is the maturing of ageing, the richness of the autumn years.

The elder has a responsibility not just to stagnate and become depressed, but to share his broader overview, his hard-earned wisdom, and so add to the collective. It is not just a drawing from the past, but a looking to the future, helping to temper the drive of the younger generation. It is to remind them that the future is not just about their future, but the future of many generations to come.

Imagine a world guided by optimistic spiritually enlightened elders, balancing enthusiasm of the younger generations. This is the challenge for the next generation of the elderly finally to wake up to their role in society. To work with optimum healing, and find their true place as wise counsellors.

Death and grief

Our greatest and final challenge is to face death. With optimum healing peace can be found for the dying, compassion given by the carers, meaning comes from the experience, and every death can be met with dignity. Death becomes a natural healing experience.

The first part of this chapter is about the basic facts of death, and the process of dying, which will help to deepen understanding. The challenge of death is faced by making practical preparations with spiritual intentions. The goal is to die in a calm and peaceful state. This is essential as it determines how the soul moves on. To be in optimum health when dying one needs to be as free as possible of all the negative attributes. Two qualities that help with dying are acceptance and forgiveness. This in turn leads to deepening spiritual awareness. Finally there is some advice for those attending the dying before the important subject of grief is addressed.

A hundred years ago in Britain three out of ten children died before reaching the age of five, and the average life expectancy was not much more than forty years old. Death was a common experience, and a frequent visitor to our communities, indiscriminately taking young and old alike. By contrast in modern times death among the young is uncommon, and many people do not experience a death of someone close to them until later in their lives.

I can remember being called by ambulance men to the house of an old man who had collapsed and died in his toilet. My job was to certify that he was dead. Shortly after, the police arrived to interview the dead man's wife. This is a legal requirement following a sudden death. Then the undertaker came to collect the body.

From the time of the man saying to his wife he was going to the toilet to being carried out of the house dead in a box, was only two hours. It was all done with cold efficiency, and gave his wife little chance to come to terms with what had happened.

Death is also feared. We seem to have forgotten how to behave when attending the dead. In modern society it is often sanitised as a means of avoiding pain. Part of the problem is simply an unfamiliarity with dying, and when death does enter our personal lives we are ill equipped to deal with it. We avoid discussing it, and if we do it is often by making jokes. However, by facing the basic facts of death, understanding the process of dying, and preparing for death, we can reduce the fear.

First it is important to be aware of three basic facts concerning death.

1 Death is inevitable

It is something we cannot escape. We cannot alter the fact by using force, bribes or wealth. Influence, power or medicines cannot stop us all dying some time. Death comes to everyone, rich or poor.

2 We cannot predict when we will die

We may hope to live to an old age, but death can strike at any age through illness or accident. The length of each life is unpredictable.

3 There is no way of extending life indefinitely

We may resort to medicines or potions, try various methods to prolong our life, but eventually we all die.

Yet many people fool themselves that death will not happen, or cannot happen to them so soon. So they put off thinking about it; they are too busy and have too many commitments to give it any serious consideration. They like to believe that their death will be in the distant future. Then when they have to face up to the reality either in themselves or in others, they are not prepared.

The purpose of considering these three basic facts is not to instil fear, but to avoid wasting our lives. It makes us appreciate what little time we have. It gives us a sense of urgency to get on with what we feel important not only to do, but with our own spiritual development.

The process of dying

There is a fear that dying must be an agonising experience, or you will lose your mind and control of bodily functions. However the reality is that most deaths are easy, peaceful events, particularly in old age, or after a long illness.

1 Physical changes at death

As the end approaches, the physical body becomes weaker, with the dying person taking less interest in food and drink. In the weeks before death he or she will generally lose weight, and in the days before death pass less urine. The muscles of the body will become weaker. Taste may diminish, but the sense of hearing and sight remain very much intact. In the hours leading up to death breathing becomes laboured.

The point of physical death is usually quite peaceful, when finally the breathing stops. If you are with someone who is dying do not be alarmed if the breathing has stopped for over a minute, and the person then takes another deep sigh. This can happen several times before finally there are no more breaths. The heartbeat will have stopped, which is the final test of death. Doctors will ascertain if death has occurred by listening to the heart with a stethoscope, or by feeling for a pulse in the neck. They will then check the eyes with a torch to test that they no longer contract to light. If that is the case the brain is beyond recovery.

The body will become stiff quite quickly, within one to two hours, so it is best to put the person in a position that is easy to move later. Usually they are laid out straight on their back, with arms at the side and feet together. It is normal to close the eyes, and prop the chin with a pillow so the mouth is closed.

It is unusual that there is incontinence of urine or faeces, but there may be some leakage after death, so it is best to have an incontinence sheet over the bed. Under normal circumstances the body may take several days before there is any sign of it decomposing. The signs of decomposition are a change in colour from the usual slight pallor of the dead person, to at first a pink, then blue, and eventually a green tinge on the skin. This change is usually first seen on the abdomen, then the chest, limbs and face. Such changes are gradual over several days. A body will not smell unless it has been left for some time. After three or four days there may begin some bloating of the body as gases are released internally. Bodies that are diseased, especially with infection, will decompose more quickly. Bodies will also decompose more quickly if they are thin, or left in a warm atmosphere. If you are leaving the body in a house for several days to view, leave him or her in the coolest room, and turn off the heating. You can always contact your local undertaker for advice.

A common practice now is for undertakers to embalm a body if it is to be viewed by relatives. This involves injecting preservative fluid into a vessel to replace some blood. The dead person will then show none of the signs of decomposition, and look much the same as they did when alive.

2 The mind at death

The mind of the dying person may lapse in and out of consciousness, but at one level is aware of everything going on. The conscious mind begins to fade before physical death. The physical senses lessen, as does memory and thinking. At another level the dying person is aware of everything around them. This is worth remembering when attending a dying person. Speak to them as though they can hear and understand everything. Even your thoughts can be picked up in such situations.

This was something I became aware of after visiting a dying patient of mine in hospital. She had not spoken for two days, and had lapsed into an unconscious state. As I held her hand I was thinking it was a pity that she and her husband had not been able to accept that she was going to die, and they would not have an opportunity to say goodbye to each other. As I sat next to her thinking about this dilemma, she raised her paralysed hand, and signalled for me to come closer. Then in a clear voice said that she knew she was dying, and now wished to say a few words to her husband. Fortunately he was in the room and was able to come to her side to hear what she had to say. She relapsed into unconsciousness again, and died peacefully the following day.

I have seen with the dying person a turning point when they seem to accept the inevitability of death, and they no longer struggle. Consequently the final days or hours are much more peaceful. The symptoms of their illness are less, and they seem to require fewer drugs. I remember such a patient with lung cancer, who although she understood she had a terminal illness and had only two to three months to live, denied that she was dying and persisted in making arrangements for the following year. She was already on strong painkillers, and needed a lot of attention from her partially disabled husband. She agreed to be admitted to a hospice to give her husband a break, and then to everyone's surprise she died two days later. It could have been said that she had 'given up'. However I feel that following admission to the hospice at some level she accepted she was going to die. She had saved herself a lot of needless suffering and further anguish to her husband who would have had to witness her gradual and painful deterioration.

3 The spirit at death

The crucial question then remains. What happens to the spirit at death? Often when attending a death there is an awareness that the person is no longer there. They have gone, departed; it is as simple as that. Some nurses who work with the dying have occasionally reported a kind of luminous blue-white light that moves away from the dead body soon after death. Is this the spirit leaving the body? Others report seeing a cord that joins the physical body break off. Is this the soul breaking free? This observation is more a subtle impression rather than seeing with the eyes.

It seems that at the point of death the spirit of the person rises out of the body, and pauses before setting off to join the greater spirit where it belongs. It moves on to, or into, another dimension. How and where we do not know. What an interesting and an exciting prospect!

The pause before finally leaving the body is probably similar to what is described as the 'near-death experience'. This is when the departing spirit views their body before moving off towards the light. For how long we do not know, as it seems that in this dimension of existence time is on a different scale.

On one occasion I was called out to a woman as an emergency in the middle of the morning surgery. Her husband had telephoned to ask for a house call as she had developed diarrhoea some hours before, and now he said she had severe abdominal pains. When I arrived at the door I was greeted by her husband saying he thought she had food poisoning, but that she was now unconscious. I rushed into the bedroom to find her dead. She had no pulses, and had stopped breathing. Her husband, who was standing by the bedroom door, asked if she would be fit enough to play in a bridge match at the weekend. I shouted to ask him to go and call for the ambulance urgently. As I stood alone with the dead woman I wondered what I would do next, and what I was going to say to the poor man. Then I noticed something on the ceiling. Something like a faint light. I did not see it with my eyes. It was more a kind of inner seeing. It was the woman's departing spirit. I thought to myself, and directed the thought to her, You had better get back into that body quickly or your husband is going to be very upset.

At that point her body gave a shudder, and she started to breathe again. The ambulance crew arrived shortly after, and the patient was taken to hospital where she was operated on for a ruptured major blood vessel. She never regained consciousness, and died one month later. Three months after that her husband came to consult me on a minor matter. As he was leaving he said, 'You know I had no idea how ill my wife was when you came to see her on that day. I needed that month of visiting her in hospital after her operation to get used to the idea that she was going to die.'

4 Emotions at death

There is another level to our being which is neither mind nor spirit. It is called the psychic field, or emotional level. This matrix of the person can be described as a print of their emotions. It may take some hours to dissolve after death, and is another reason to allow the body to settle before moving it. On rare occasions it can last for months or even years, especially if the dead person has had a disturbed life or death, and is felt as a cold atmosphere in the area.

A **doctor friend was** converting an old house into a surgery. In one of the rooms things always seemed to go wrong. Tools would get lost, lights would not work, fittings would fall down. They noticed it was always cold in one corner. It became so bad that the workmen would no longer work in the room. Then one of the receptionists who was particularly sensitive felt the presence of an old lady. When enquiries were made it was discovered the previous owner's elderly mother had died in that room ten years before. A simple little ceremony to clear the space removed her remaining psychic/emotional matrix, and they never had any more trouble.

Sudden death

When death occurs suddenly one does not have the opportunity to go through the gradual process as outlined above. The physical and mental processes cease abruptly, and the spiritual essence leaves the body. The emotional field may remain for some time as I described, and for that reason it is best not to move the body, but for practical reasons, such as the safety of others, it may have to be moved. As far as possible the same spiritual awareness should be observed as outlined for a natural death.

Practical preparations, spiritual intentions

1 Make a will: acceptance

Deciding to make a will is a good first step in preparing for your own death. At least it is an admission that you are going to die, and does give you a chance to reflect how those left behind will manage without you. In this country it is said that 30 per cent of people who die have not made a will. Any lawyer will tell you that a clear list of how possessions are to be distributed prevents endless squabbling.

There is no time to lose if you have not yet made a will, as death can occur unexpectedly. It is not an expensive thing to do, and is usually quite straightforward. Once done, you have begun to accept your own death.

2 Clear the decks: release

It is important to keep your finances and documents up to date. Check life insurance, and other provisions you may have made for your loved ones. As you get older, and death is more likely, it is worth having an annual clear-out of all unnecessary possessions. They can be given away to friends or charities, which gives a feeling of freedom. It is an idea to give some of your treasured valuables to relatives and friends now, which does have the merit that they have an opportunity to thank you. My own mother has put coloured stickers on all her possessions so everyone knows who is getting what. She has given away most of her jewellery to her grandchildren, which gave her the pleasure of seeing them appreciate something that meant so much to her.

This physical act of sorting out our possessions and letting them go helps to prepare for the inevitably more difficult breaking of emotional and spiritual ties that comes with death.

3 Arrange your funeral: lightness

Making arrangements for your own funeral is another way of acknowledging that death can happen at any time. Addressing such practical issues involved in organising a funeral does encourage us to face the reality of our own physical mortality.

Do you wish to be buried or cremated? What type of funeral service or coffin do you want? Is the service to be in a church, or somewhere else? Would you like certain hymns sung or poems read, and would you like flowers, or a collection for charity? Would you like your body left for research? This may sound unduly morbid, but it certainly frees the survivors from worry at a time when they may find making decisions difficult.

Mr Rowan had a major bowel operation, and had been sent home by the hospital because there was nothing left to be done. I was shocked at his poor condition, and doubted he would survive the weekend. It was necessary to outline to him quite frankly what was happening so that he could complete any arrangements he needed to make with his relatives. Only when I explained to him the seriousness of his situation did I realise that he had no idea about his condition. He had spent the previous months in ignorance and fear. Now that he knew the worst, in his typically down-to-earth way he could get on with it, making all the practical arrangements for his funeral. Much to my surprise, and that of his relatives, he began to improve, and within two months was driving his car again. He lived for a further year, dying shortly after attending his granddaughter's marriage. In Mr Rowan's case arranging his funeral led to an immediate improvement in well-being, and a prolongation of life, but this cannot be guaranteed in every case!

The fear of the unknown is always worse than the reality. Once faced with the facts it does not sound so gruesome. You have to do more than just think about these questions, but make decisions and leave specific instructions. Many funeral directors welcome people to discuss the details of their work.

4 Write a eulogy, epitaph and story: reflection and completion

Writing a piece to be read at your funeral is another way of preparing for death. Some people write their own obituaries to be published after they have died. What would you like written on your tombstone as an epitaph?

Resting in peace. At peace at last. Lived serving others. Now flying free.

A more private exercise is to write the story of your life, which can have the added purpose of reviewing your life to date. It does give you a chance to complete some things that have been left unfinished, or to take up others that you always wished to have done.

5 Be interested in death: understanding

This is not to suggest that you develop some kind of morbid preoccupation with death but concerning ourselves with death when it does appear in our lives, and not avoiding it, is a means of preparing for our own death. We can do this by simply trying to understand how the bereaved must feel, and respond to their needs appropriately. Besides being involved with the situation, at the same time we can stand back and observe ourselves. Then we can learn from our own feelings, and how we cope with them.

6 Visualising death: facing the fear

Preparing for death can be done by imagining your own death. How do you see yourself dying? Suddenly in an accident, or in your own bed? From a heart attack or after a long illness?

It can be difficult to imagine yourself on your deathbed surrounded by loved ones and saying goodbye for the last time. Imagine how you would look and how you would feel. It is certainly worth doing as an exercise as, if repeated, the fear will gradually become less.

When do you think you will die? In your eighties, seventies, sixties or much younger? What would you do if you only had six months to live?

Embracing positive qualities

Acceptance

This quality has been already mentioned but is worth emphasising again, as the need to accept death as inevitable at a deep spiritual level allows for an easy death. I have seen religious believers, including priests, who have struggled at their deaths because of the fear. This may be because their faith was based on teachings, and it was not something they had experienced and integrated into their heart.

Adrian was one of those patients we as carers found particularly difficult. He was forty-one years old, and had terminal lung cancer. He maintained that he was thinking positively about his cancer by believing he was going to recover. He would not accept the possibility of his death, and visited many specialist centres seeking various treatments. It was distressing for his family as they had no chance to prepare and say goodbye. His pain control was difficult as he had a fear of dying in his sleep, and fought against his medication. The patience of the nurses was rewarded when in his final day he accepted the inevitable, and bade his farewells before slipping into his first and last restful sleep.

Before beginning to think positively, one first needs to accept the situation. This applies to illness and to death.

An old farmer I remember well told me a few days before his death that he had last been in a church as a child when someone threw water in his face when he was christened. But that same man made a point each day of getting up to see the sun rise, and would sit quietly to watch it slip down behind the hill of his farmhouse each day. When he died he slipped away himself as naturally and as peacefully as the sun setting.

Forgiveness

Letting go of past grudges and practising forgiveness in the days before death is an important way of clearing the mind.

Over the years people may have offended us or hurt us in a way that is difficult to forgive. Yet this is an important task that we must carry out. We can only die at peace if we are free of all the negative qualities. As we do not know when we may die, it is best to begin to address any of these negative feelings we have for others now.

Think of people whom you hold resentments against, or you feel have wronged you in the past, and hold them in your mind. Then, as sincerely as possible, forgive them from your heart. Remember also to forgive yourself, for things you perhaps did not achieve, or perhaps things you wished you had said. After all, you may have done your best at the time. Even if you had not, the feelings of regret now serve no purpose, and one should let them go and free yourself.

An **eighteen-year-old** college student was at first devastated to learn he was HIV positive, and his recent illness was indeed AIDS. After professional counselling he was able to 'come out' concerning his homosexuality. He told his parents and friends, and dealt with all their initial hostility towards him. Knowing he had at the most two years to live, he realised he only had a limited time left to develop himself spiritually and prepare for his death. Before, he had been uncertain about his future, but appreciating the little time left he embarked on a photographic career. He accepted that he was going to die, and felt he could forgive everyone their past prejudices. His philosophy became to live very much for the present. He helped with an AIDS charity himself, and despite showing physical deterioration after each relapse, spiritually one could see him grow. He positively radiated a zest for life. He lived for eighteen months from his diagnosis and died very peacefully.

Attending the dying person

With the experience gained from the hospice movement in recent years patients should no longer fear they will suffer from any physical discomfort as a result of a terminal illness. Health care workers are well trained to give the kind of attention and care needed by the patient, but much can also be done by friends and relatives.

If you are involved in caring for someone dying, such as a relative or friend, you can really help them if you are at ease with your own death. Facing death is probably the biggest challenge of our life, and it seems foolish not to be prepared. It should no longer be viewed as a fight against a foe, as it is one battle that we will inevitably lose, but seen as a challenge, which is a final healing.

Companionship

When a child is born it is welcomed with love by the parents. Everyone is joyful about the new arrival. In the same way when a person dies those in attendance should send them off with love and good wishes on their final journey.

Everyone involved in the care of the dying person needs not only to be acting with kindness, but thinking loving thoughts. No matter how well prepared the dying person is, they are having to face up to the reality of death. This is when they need a companion on their last challenge in this life.

There will be times when the dying person will wish to share their fears and worries about death and dying. It may well be that the person they choose happens to be you. The best thing a good friend can do is to listen. If they ask questions, answer them as honestly as you can. It is not the time to begin to preach your spiritual ideas. Be there for them with your full attention. Make some time, and just sit and listen. Such listening is a precious gift you can give them as a friend. Listen with an open mind without making any judgement.

Those closest to the dying person can be the object of their anger and resentment. You may be the one in the firing line. Do not take it personally. They may well be feeling alone and afraid, and it is their way of expressing such fear. Keep foremost in your mind thoughts of love towards that person. One way of doing this is to think of happy times you shared together.

Creating peace

In the days preceding death the dying person needs to be at peace, and every attempt should be made by those caring for them to make this possible. Those caring for the dying person need to be calm and relaxed. They should show no fear, and be reassuring that dying is an easy process. If relatives are present they should not express their grief in front of them in the days before death. The room they are nursed in, whether in hospital or at home, should be quiet and peaceful. The decoration should be simple, using soft pastel shades, and perhaps some flowers. There should be no distractions to remind the dying person of what they may be leaving behind.

Eric was dying from a stroke, and his wife cried for long periods beside his bed. I had to remind her not to express her emotions so fully in front of him in his last days. She had nursed him at home on her own for two years, and now after another stroke he was gradually slipping away. Her crying, although necessary for herself, did not allow him the chance to find the calmness that he required.

If at all possible one's grief should be expressed away from the bedside. The dying person should not be troubled with matters of this world, and that includes the emotions of others. They need to focus on preparing themselves for their transition.

Helping the departed soul

On the spiritual level thinking of the dead person in a positive way, and invoking a prayer or a dedication will help them on their journey. If we do believe the soul is eternal, their existence continues after death, so our thoughts do have an influence.

After physical death the soul may have left the body but it may have some way to travel before it reaches its final resting place. That is why the onus is on those left to help the spiritual part on its journey by being as positive and accepting as possible. This is especially important in a sudden death, as a longing for the dead person may disorientate the departing spirit on its journey. This does not mean one should not grieve, but the intention is to allow the departing soul to reach his or her destination in peace.

After a death a common feeling is to wish you could do something. I do not mean in this instance to regret you had not done something to have saved the dead person, but you could do something now. Giving a gift to their favourite charity, or supporting some project that has a spiritual aim is one way of doing something on behalf of the person who has passed over.

Negative experience

If you have experienced the death of a loved one and failed to carry out any of these suggestions, do not look back with regret. We gain nothing thinking about missed opportunities; what we can do, though, is learn from them. Do not use the phrase 'if only' but look forward and consider how your experience can benefit others. Start by thinking what would have helped you in your own situation. If you know of someone in a similar situation you may have the opportunity to advise them. Remember it is not the loud voice of the convert that is listened to, but the quiet word said at the appropriate moment that has the most effect. Things have a strange way of working out for the best if your intention is for the best. If you do have some advice or experience to give to others somehow people who need such advice are attracted to you. Watch and be attentive, and you can help others having yourself learned through mistakes. After all, we all make mistakes, but it is the spiritual person who learns from these mistakes who can benefit his or her fellow man.

Grieving

Some time in our lives, sooner or later we are all going to lose a loved one. It could be a parent, a child, a friend, a husband or wife. They might die suddenly, or after a period of illness. Few escape the experience of grief. It is a worthwhile task to try to understand what is normal grief to prepare us for this challenge.

Typically following a death the first reaction is shock and denial. This soon leads on to sorrow and anguish. There may be anger, guilt, and even relief. The low point comes with the full realisation of the loss, the feeling of hopelessness, isolation and depression. But gradually with time we adapt to the change, and learn acceptance. The whole process of grieving then becomes healing.

The pattern of grieving is partially determined by the culture we live in and our own family traditions. Some societies have fixed periods of grieving lasting so many days or months. There may be traditions that the bereaved are expected to conform to, such as wearing black clothes. In certain communities it is not acceptable to be seen enjoying oneself for the period of one year, and out of respect for the dead some activities are avoided, or abstinence of certain foods is practised.

I have seen in Africa, where death is a common visitor, anguish being expressed by the bereaved in the extreme. The relatives and friends take to loud wailing, screeching, beating of chests, and throwing themselves to the ground in uncontrollable distress. This intense expression of anguish can go on for several days. It may be a matter of survival for them to have such an extreme experience as it enables them quickly to return to their daily tasks.

The experience of mourning is variable and can be totally preoccupying and overwhelming. One can feel quite all right, only in the next moment to be overcome with powerful thoughts and emotions. The intensity fluctuates throughout the whole grieving process.

Mr Johnson was a bank manager whose wife died of breast cancer. Two weeks after the funeral he returned to work and everything carried on much as before. When he visited the surgery he would cry uncontrollably for most of the consultation. He said he cried occasionally at home, but never in front of anyone. He commented that he always felt better after. His appointments at the surgery became less frequent over the weeks, and one day six months after his wife's death he announced he no longer needed to come and see me. It was not because he had 'got over it', but in the last months his neighbours had been very kind, and he felt he could now turn to them for support.

The length of grieving is also quite variable, but two years could be described as normal following the loss of someone close.

Mrs Foster asked for an anti-depressant drug as she still felt tearful and depressed two months after her husband's death. She said that her friends and family had been so supportive to her that she felt guilty as she was such poor company. When I explained that the average time taken for the whole grieving process is between six months to two years, she was surprised and relieved. I went on to say that over this time she could expect to have good, and not so good, days. The suffering would gradually become less intense, and the happy memories of the time they spent together would become clearer.

I find that it is extremely common for patients to consult their general practitioner with all kinds of conditions following a bereavement.

Margaret in the year following her husband's death visited the surgery with a multitude of different complaints including itchy skin, poor sleep, tiredness, joint aches and outbursts of crying. Then one day she announced at the end of the consultation she was going to visit her husband's grave for the first time as it was the anniversary of his death. She felt it would mark the end of her grieving. Her consultations thereafter were much less, and many of her complaints diminished.

Grieving not only applies in death, it can be any loss in our lives, large or small. It can be the loss of a job, loss of a pet, loss of a limb, loss of home, loss of nationality, or loss of a relationship such as through divorce.

Janet's forty-year-old son was involved in a car accident, and he was left not only with a physical disability, but mentally he became a very difficult person. She had to grieve not only for the lost personality of her son, but for all the hopes she had had for him. Besides the hard work of looking after him, she had to grieve for her own loss of the hopes she had had for her own retirement.

The five aspects to grieving

Grieving is a healing process, and is essentially a spiritual experience. There are five aspects of grieving, which I will look at in some detail. Remember that each aspect is normal and natural. These are:

1   Denial
2   Sorrow
3   Negative qualities: anger
                            worry
                            attachment

1 Denial

Denial is quite a normal reaction. Very often immediately after a death the recently bereaved will return to the body several times in disbelief to check that he or she really is dead. There is a numbness, almost as if all thinking and feeling functions are frozen. It is described as 'being in shock', and can last for hours or days.

Mrs Yates and her husband had returned from a walk together, and as he had some stomach pains he went to lie down. When she went to wake him for dinner he was dead. She tried for half an hour to rouse him before contacting me as his doctor. Even when I confirmed that he was dead, she did not believe it, and persisted in shaking him to wake him up. An old friend whose own husband had died suddenly some years before was at hand to comfort her. She stayed with her during those difficult several hours.

Denial is a mechanism we use to adapt to a sudden change. The implications of someone dying who is close to us are enormous, and it is no wonder that we try to pretend it has not happened. Denial is an essential process to lessen the pain, and helps us to deal with the immediate practical arrangements that have to be made.

After the initial period of denial, one begins to accept the physical reality of the new situation. Doing practical things such as informing relatives, and arranging for the body to be moved helps to come to terms with the situation. But doubts can return as to whether the person has really died. Even after the funeral further thoughts of denial are common, and certainly not abnormal. Thoughts that perhaps it was all a dream, and we will soon wake up, or that the person has gone away on holiday and it did not really happen.

I can remember visiting a lady whose husband had died three hours before I arrived at her house. She refused to make any arrangements about moving him, as she said her husband was still alive. They had been married for fifty-five years. When together we looked at his body she of course knew he was dead, but continued to tell me he was just asleep. It was the following day before she finally got round to contacting the undertaker.

It does take time to integrate a change, and denial is a mechanism for doing it gradually. It is only when this denial continues that it blocks the person's normal function.

Young children may have a different aspect of denial, especially if grieving for someone close such as a parent. Despite being told of the parent's death, they repeatedly will ask where their parent is, and go to look for them. I have seen this type of pining for a lost loved one in elderly patients too.

I n one instance a lady in her eighties called me to visit because she thought her sister, whom she had lived with, had been missing for two weeks. Actually she had died six months previously. When I talked to her she readily agreed she was dead, and could discuss the details of her sister's funeral. At the same time she was worried that her sister did not have her medication with her while she was away. She was not demented at all, and managed her normal household chores quite adequately. This form of denial was her method of adapting to the loss of her sister who was her close lifelong companion. Listening and talking helped.

2 Sorrow

Sorrow is the central experience of grief. It arises from the sense of loss, which we all have gone through at some time. Even when it is a temporary misplacement, like the car keys, it can be preoccupying. The loss of a loved one can be agonising and intense. Sorrow hurts. It is pain. It can make one want to cry out in despair at the helplessness and hopelessness of the situation. What had meaning in our life no longer seems to have meaning. It has an emptiness to it, like falling into a dark hole.

Mrs Hide's husband died at fifty-five, and she felt completely bereft. They had no children and through their thirty years together had shared many common interests. Her sorrow was difficult to bear. She cried for long periods, and felt very alone. Her life was now empty. Two months after his death she came to the surgery with a list of physical symptoms: headaches, poor appetite, chest aches, joint pains and difficulty with sleep. Her mental symptoms included racing thoughts, difficulty with concentration, poor memory. Emotionally she was flat and irritable. Spiritually one could say she was sad and lonely.

She told me that her employers were sympathetic, so she was able to stay off work for some months. When she did return many people were supportive towards her, and encouraged her to go out with them. A year after his death she reported she began to feel better, and after eighteen months many of her symptoms had improved. She could begin to see some future for herself. Not only is time a great healer, but so is human companionship.

Mr Roland found a different quality to alleviate his sorrow. It had been four years since his wife's death, and now his own health was beginning to deteriorate with heart failure. Until then he had been an active eighty-four-year-old, but now found he could no longer manage because of his breathlessness. I sent him into hospital because of his worsening condition, and when I visited him at home after his discharge he looked surprisingly well. I remarked on this, and he said the laughter and cheerfulness of the young nurses had lifted his spirits. He realised that he did not have much time left to live himself, and had resolved to be as cheerful as possible, and this cheerfulness was the quality that was to help him resolve his grief.

Sorrow can be likened to a wound. It hurts, is painful and can bleed. And like a wound if it is left it can fester. It needs to be attended to and protected, and allowed to heal at its own natural rate. The rate of healing will in turn depend on the state of the rest of the body. Like a wound it will leave a scar, but that doesn't necessarily mean it deforms the rest of the body.

The hurting feeling of sorrow can lead the individual to look for some kind of cause for this feeling. They may wish to blame someone and seek revenge. However real that may seem, it is a spiritual cul-de-sac. It is best to accept sorrow as an intrinsic part of life (which it is) like any other emotion or feeling, and make the best of it. Do not blame others, or even yourself. If that feeling does arise think of the spiritual quality of forgiveness. Think about the circumstances and the people involved, and either to yourself or out loud say that you forgive them. In that way you grow spiritually out of the experience.

Different cultures deal with sorrow in their own way. In Europe the people of the northern countries tend to control their emotions, whereas peoples of the southern Mediterranean countries show them. They cry more openly to express their deep hurt and loss. Tears are a way of acknowledging feelings, and enable people to move from a passive state of sadness and emptiness into a more active state of being. It gives one energy to move on. Too much control of emotions can lead to a damming-up of feelings which need releasing. They fester, only to come out later as illness. On the other hand too much crying may lead to complete emotional exhaustion. As always it is a matter of balance, and doing what is appropriate for you in your own setting. It is what feels right for each person as an individual. There is no right or wrong way to express sorrow.

The emptiness of sorrow is sometimes described as being in a dark prison cell compared to a beautiful countryside. All the colour, smells, shapes and movement have gone and one is left with nothing. The rich tapestry of life seems meaningless. It is bland, pointless, monotonous. The present is black. The prospects for the future seem empty, and even making plans and decisions needs a great effort.

'It is best to keep busy,' may seem grossly inappropriate to the situation, but there is some truth to it. Keeping in touch with the routine tasks of life helps. To the recently bereaved it may seem pointless, but they are important strands to begin to reconnect with the mainstream of life again.

3 Negative qualities

All the five negative qualities, anger, worry, attachment, guilt and depression, are seen in grieving, commonly when they are found to be the root cause of illness after a death or loss.

ANGER

It is common to feel anger after a death. Anger with ourselves for not being considerate enough towards the dead person, and angry with the person for dying. Anger is not usually considered as appropriate following a death, and tends to be suppressed, eventually to show itself as illness.

Mrs Wilson had a persistent and long-standing ache in her shoulders. Towards the end of one consultation I asked her what she thought made her symptoms worse. She said it was the stress of being on her own, and having to cope with difficult neighbours. But she went on to say the pains really started twelve years previously, shortly after her husband's death. She had nursed him through a long and difficult illness, and felt angry that such a good man should die when there are so many bad people in the world. She felt angry that nothing more could have been done, and was angry with him for leaving her on her own. Undoubtedly this anger was the cause of her physical problem.

Often at the receiving end of the anger of the grieving person are those who were involved with the medical care of the dead person. Doctors, nurses, physiotherapists, chaplains and caring relatives are the targets for this anger.

The anger can be directed at the 'dead person' for being inconsiderate, and leaving them behind to manage on their own. As it is not usually acceptable to admit to anger in this context it is tinged with guilt.

The same is true when people are angry at God for taking their loved one away. There can be a feeling of being let down, as if in some way we merit special treatment from God for being good. What anger does do in this situation is that it ultimately challenges our relationship with God.

Mrs Bachelor came to see me with what appeared to be a fairly routine complaint of a pain in her knee after a fall. I explained it could take over eight weeks for her knee to get better, and she would have to be off work. She seemed angry with the suggestion, and said that she could not afford to be off work, as she was the wage-earner in the family. She continued, with tears in her eyes, to tell me how shortly after the birth of her daughter her husband had died of leukemia. They had been so looking forward to family life, and she still felt angry that she was denied that happiness and had to go out to work. The knee injury, and its consequences, brought up some of the old anger concerning her husband's death. When she did begin to express the anger it was directed at God because she felt she had been treated so unfairly.

Guidelines to deal with anger are outlined in the chapter on anger. The key elements are: first of all be responsible for the anger, and do not project it on to other people; then reflect why you are angry; go on to evaluate whether that anger is appropriate, especially at a time when you are so upset. Ultimately it is a question of forgiveness and tolerance of ourselves, and then of others.

WORRY

Mrs Wilmott is a thirty-six-year-old dental receptionist. Her initial complaint was a sore dry throat, and choking sensation which had started two weeks before. Having examined her and told her there was little physically wrong, she said it must be worry, as she is normally very fit. She had more worries than usual, such as selling her house. But what had upset her most was the death of her young dog three weeks previously. She had not expressed her grief to anyone, and only by talking she realised it was connected to her anxiety symptoms. This realisation that there was a causal link with her symptoms and the dog's death soon resulted in the sore throat and choking symptoms going.

Incidentally, one could speculate that the choking was a difficulty in swallowing the fact that her dog had died.

Another case of worry associated with grief was that of a lady whose symptoms, two years after her husband's death, if anything were getting worse. She would wake up at night in a panic worrying about all the previous day's events, and then worry about the next day. She constantly thought of her dead husband. Trying to rid herself of such thoughts she found difficult. Rather than try to rid herself of her racing thoughts, I suggested it might be helpful if she wrote all her concerns down as if in a letter to her husband. After several such letters, she had the idea of also writing the reply for him.

This exercise helped her express her worries, and see them for what they were. They were just thoughts. She began to sleep better, and one day some years later she told me she had written a final goodbye letter to her husband.

ATTACHMENT

Once the person is dead we have to learn to let go our physical attachment. To let go the emotional attachment too can be much harder.

Mrs Dawson was such a case. She had not consulted me for many years, but then presented with a mixture of symptoms including swollen neck glands, numbness of her fingers, weakness, weight loss and feeling depressed. Urgent investigations at the hospital failed to find a cause. Meanwhile her condition deteriorated, and her only relative, a niece, came to discuss her future care. She was able to tell me that her aunt's symptoms had started after her husband's death the previous year. They had no children, and she described her aunt as a stubborn person who was completely dependent on her husband emotionally. Her aunt was very resentful about his death, and could not move beyond this feeling. The niece was sure that was why she was ill. Before we could arrange further nursing care the old lady died in hospital.

Couples can become very dependent upon each other's support almost to the exclusion of others. When one partner dies, the remaining spouse has no one to confide in, or share their feelings with. By examining now, in the present, the kind of attachment we have towards our loved ones, and they to us, we can begin to lessen the blow when one of us dies.

Mrs Stanford was another case of emotional attachment. She was a bit of a recluse, and her husband had died two years previously. She told me that she could see her husband every evening lingering by the curtains in the lounge and often spoke to him. She felt a bit annoyed as he did not seem to want to be there, but she felt some comfort in seeing him. However she was concerned that she might be going mad having these hallucinations. I was able to reassure her that she was not going mad, and to see such figures is quite common. It is not the physical body that one sees, but a kind of emotional template of the departed person. We talked some more about this figure, and she began to understand that he himself wanted to move on. It was her own emotional need that was holding him back. For her own sake, and his, she had to break the emotional chain. Only then would they both be free.

Part of loving someone, alive or dead, is letting go and giving them the freedom to move on. That was what Mrs Stanford had to do: say to the figure of her husband that she was releasing him on his journey, and that she could now manage on her own. Reluctantly she agreed, and when I saw her again some months later she told me how difficult it had been, but she now realised it had been the right thing to do.

Use the following exercise by asking in what way you are physically dependent on those close to you. Ask yourself how could you manage the simple tasks of housekeeping, cooking, shopping, paying the bills, changing an electric plug, etc., without the other person. Then consider what emotional demands you make on them, which perhaps limit them, and how dependent emotionally you are on them. Do we only offer our love when they conform to our needs? Is this love tinged with selfishness, envy and jealousy?

The only attachment that can remain is spiritual, and that is love. That love is free of possessiveness. It is wanting what is best for that person, and is not dependent on what we need. When death comes, as it surely will, with love the parting is easier, and the love survives. What the departed soul really wishes of those left behind is for the bereaved to continue to think of them in a positive light. They would also want them to recover from their grief quickly, and continue with their own life plan.

Only by looking at our attachment today can we develop this true unselfish love, and free ourselves of the physical and emotional needs we demand of others. We can then appreciate their positive aspects, and that gives them encouragement to grow spiritually. Such an attitude will only serve to strengthen the relationship.

The end of each day is a kind of death. It is a good exercise just to spend a few moment before you go to sleep thinking back over the day. The good moments, and perhaps some problems you have had to face. The mistakes made, and how you can learn from them. Give thanks, which allows us to move on to the next day. By practising this each day eventually the partings at death will be less painful.

GUILT

Guilt is experienced by most people during mourning. We were not there when we felt we should have been. We remember things that we said or did, or did not say or do, and then feel guilty. It is common to have a sense of relief that the person has now gone, especially if the deceased had a long illness. That seems such a selfish thought, then there are feelings of guilt.

Mrs Daniels was having a routine blood pressure check when she mentioned that her diamond wedding anniversary was the previous week. There was a certain sadness in her voice, and she went on to explain that it reminded her of her only daughter who had died fifteen years before of leukemia. She felt guilty about not saying goodbye to her properly, and resentful towards the staff at the hospital who prevented her seeing her body. She and her husband never talked about it now, but the feelings always arose at anniversaries. She felt she needed to talk some more on the subject, and resolved to talk to a good friend at her local bridge club who she knew to be a good listener.

Inevitably we blame ourselves for not having done enough around the time of death, or during the deceased person's life. These thoughts are bound to arise, but there is nothing to be gained by holding on to them. This self-punishment will only make us feel worse. Even if you believe it to be true, you need to forgive yourself with the understanding that it has been a lesson you have learned from.

Preventing guilt A way of preventing guilt or at least minimising the feelings of guilt after someone's death is to act now. Think of all those people you do love, and if they died today, in what way would you feel guilty, or feel regrets? Can you think of something that you wish you had said to that person? Perhaps it is something quite simple like to thank them, or say that you love and appreciate them. You may have wanted to give them a present, or simply to compliment them. Bring yourself up to date, and do it at the first suitable opportunity.

DEPRESSION

With grief there are two types of depression. The first is a normal adaptive process. It is withdrawing into ourselves to give us time and space to reflect. It is a necessary period of quiet to slow down physically, mentally and emotionally. We may seem unresponsive and detached to other people, but we do need that space in our life to deal with these strong new feelings and thoughts. Concentration may be poor for previously simple tasks, and it may be difficult to pay attention for any length of time.

Each of us needs to be sensitive to the person who has suffered a bereavement and recognise that there are times when they need quiet, and times when they need activity. Just sitting with them without any conversation is a comfort.

The other type of depression is a reaction to this deep sense of loss. It is not only the person that you have lost, but all the things that they represent to you. In the case of a married couple their whole status and position will change. It takes time to adapt to a new way. During this time features of depression are common, and can occupy the person through most of the day. In this situation people do need company and support from their relatives and friends. They need to be encouraged to look forward with hope. But a depression following a bereavement can be severe, and thoughts of suicide are not uncommon. If that is the case professional advice should be sought.

4 Loneliness

After the tears, the distress, the denial, the anger, the resentment and depression, the person bereaved is often left feeling lonely. Loneliness is that empty feeling as if something is permanently missing. Something has been lost and can never be found again. Its very permanence is like a life sentence. Loneliness, of all the feelings in grief, is the one that can last the longest, even up to the person's own death.

Some of the solutions are very obvious and quite practical. That is getting out to meet people. Even at first if it is just to go to the shops. Seeing people and making human contact makes one feel less isolated. Then take up those offers by friends to call on them. They will know how difficult it can be to pick up old contacts, particularly if you have lost a partner and are not used to going out on your own.

With loneliness we tend to become very self-centred and concerned with our own well-being. One way to overcome this is to make a point of going out to help others less fortunate than oneself. However bad your own situation is there is always someone else worse off. Being of service to others is a very positive step to getting involved in the mainstream of life again.

At another level it can be difficult to overcome loneliness as there may be a feeling that to give up grieving in some way is a betrayal of the dead person. Some of the following exercises may be helpful.

DEALING WITH LONELINESS

1 Describe the loneliness Where is it: your head, stomach, chest? What does it feel like: cold, wet, numb? What colour is it: grey, red, black?

It is even worth while trying to draw, paint, or sculpt the loneliness. Often people will describe the loneliness as a dark empty hole. In this situation it is best to try to see the hole in one's mind's eye, and then try to feel what it is like to be in such a hole.

What do you experience in your physical body when you imagine you are in this hole? It can feel very real and be terrible, but as you stay with the feeling it will begin to change. Allow this to happen, because there is a part of you that wants to change.

2 Remembering It is natural and helpful to look back on the life of someone who has died. To review their contribution as though gathering material for a biography. Like any story, besides a beginning and a middle, it now has an end. There will be the highlights of their achievements and contributions in this story. Looking back, we will have particular personal memories that we would wish to cherish. Then the positive qualities that they brought, and how that helped others. We may have feelings of regret ourselves as to our part played in their story, wishing we had said something or done something for the person who is now dead, and it is too late. As time passes we will remember more of the good times. Even early on in a bereavement it is helpful to encourage others to remember the good and positive aspects of the deceased's character. Remember the happy times spent together, the fun times, their positive qualities, their skills and so on.

If a person dies before their time we may feel that they never had the opportunity to fulfil their potential or to complete their story. Who knows the answer to these eternal questions? But it does serve to remind each of us that life is frail. It is as well to consider that any of us could die at any time. We could get a serious illness or have an accident tomorrow. If it happens to others, it could happen to us, or a loved one.

Time may be short so if there are things to say or to do, we should not waste any time and get on with the story that we sense is ours. Also we should not put too much store in the future, and believe that some time things will be better. We need to begin to start making it better now. The way to do that is to start with ourselves. It may not be possible financially, but it costs nothing to have a positive, generous and tolerant attitude. These are the spiritual qualities that we can bring into our lives at no cost to ourselves. They can only bring benefit to ourselves and everyone around us.

5 Acceptance

A death can shatter our view of the world. What previously had meaning no longer has. The person who has died may have been central to our life, the focus of attention and love. Now they have gone there is a huge gap.

There will be a point when we need to accept the loss, adjust to the change, and find a new sense of purpose. This can only be reached by fully experiencing the grief, the sorrow, the anger, the guilt, the depression, the loneliness. Indeed the whole long difficult process of grief. It is a challenge, and perhaps the most difficult one spiritually we have to face.

Acceptance comes with understanding. There are two pillars of that understanding: knowledge and wisdom. Knowledge is gained through learning. We can read about death, and learn about grieving from others, imagining how we would manage in their circumstances. We gain wisdom when we not only have experienced grief, but are awake to the experience, accepting the suffering, and searching for meaning.

It is hard to endure some of the feelings, but if we try not to bury them, we may gain some wisdom. We will emerge a more centred, stronger and perhaps a more tolerant person.

Susan, a twenty-six-year-old bank clerk, came for advice about a bald patch that was getting bigger on her head. When we discussed possible causes she could see it was due to her grief following her mother's death. Five months previously she had died suddenly of a heart attack. Her mother had been the sole carer for her own elderly parents, and now it was Susan's responsibility to look after them. An added problem was that her own father was disabled, and her only sister who could have helped had moved overseas with her husband. However, through all this she was surprised to find that she could call on an inner strength to carry her through this difficult time. She also began to see that maintaining her own health was central to the health of those she cared for. She organised some help in the evenings so she had time to herself. I was delighted when she returned six months later to show me that her hair was now fully returned. She saw that the regrowth of her hair symbolised the growth she had made herself. She had suffered, survived, and thrived.

Grief moves us out of our individually centred world, and into a place where some fundamental spiritual questions are presented.

- What is the meaning of death?
- Why did that person have to die?
- What was the purpose of their life, if any?

That may lead on to questioning ourselves.

- When will I die, and what is my purpose in life?

Keeping pets is a particularly good learning experience for children as they not only learn to care for their animals, but have to deal with their deaths.

can remember with my own children when our first hamster died. They were at first very angry with the cat for getting into the poor hamster's cage, and then with me for not making it strong enough. They would go to check if it was really dead, and stroke it. Each of the children wrote a letter to the dead hamster and collected flowers to place in an ice-cream carton where the hamster was laid out in cotton wool. Finally after two days I was instructed to dig a grave at the bottom of the garden. In the pouring rain we said a few words each about the departed animal. Tears were shed, and we turned our backs on the grave. It did not end there, as several weeks later I had to dig up the now quite decomposed corpse so that they could inspect the skeleton. This was all without any initiative from myself or my wife. How we adults can learn from children! They had created their own ritual as a way of coming to terms with the hamster's death.

It is important to tell children, whatever their age, in simple language that the person has died and is not coming back. Feelings should be shared and accepted. They should be included as part of the family in the rituals surrounding death.

By learning to deal with small everyday losses, it will help us to deal with the bigger challenge of the loss through death of a loved one. Even saying goodbye to someone for a short time is a kind of loss.

Mrs Fastnet is a remarkable lady who owns the local post office. I was called to the house the afternoon her husband collapsed in the front lounge. I attempted resuscitation, and failed in front of the whole family. When she realised that he was dead she shed her tears, then turned her attention to comforting the rest of the family. She and her husband were both Methodists, and had clear ideas about life and what happened after death. She bore no regrets and had no anger, and fully accepted the situation.

She had come to her own understanding of what death meant, and when it arrived in her own house, albeit unexpectedly, she took it as part of the whole experience of life. Two weeks after the funeral the post office reopened, and everyone got her usual welcoming smile. In her own quiet way she became an example to the whole village.

There is an inevitable cycle to everything in nature. The day starts with the sun rising and moving across the sky to sink below the other side of the horizon. Then, following night, the whole process starts again. The year has its rhythm of seasons, as does everything in nature. Every living thing has its own cycle of birth, growth, decay, and death. We are part of nature, and there are no exceptions. Rich and famous people of the past have all died, and so must we and all our loved ones too. We need to submit to, and accept, this fact. In doing so it can free us from the fear of death, and enable us to live fuller and happier lives.

This may seem all very obvious, but the major thrust of modern medicine is to fight the battle against death. There is a notion that if we can overcome illness and the natural ageing process, death will one day be denied. But meantime the battle goes on. This attitude denies a patient the opportunity to come to terms with his or her own mortality, and so die with dignity in a peaceful frame of mind.

A person who has been on the path of optimum healing will die at peace with themselves and the world. They will have released all the negative qualities, faced up to the challenges in life of illness, accidents, change and old age, and will feel in balance and whole as they pass over to the next adventure.

Recovery plan for grief

1 Understanding

That all the physical symptoms and feelings of grief are part of the normal process. You are not alone; many people have suffered the loss of loved ones, and come through the experience.

2 Being alone

You will need time and space to reflect on what has happened, and to deal with all the feelings that arise.

3 Forgiveness

Use the quality of forgiveness to overcome guilt, resentment and regret.

4 Care for yourself

Eat regularly, and get some exercise every day. Carry on with routine tasks, even if they seem pointless, as they keep you in touch with life. Renew old interests, and find new ones.

5 Remember

It is good to think back over all the happy times you spent together, and to mark anniversaries as before.

6 Changes

Do not make any immediate changes, such as moving house. You have had one major change in your life with a death, and having another just adds further stress. Wait until you feel you have got over your grief.

7 Companionship

Welcome friends who wish to help although at times their presence may seem inappropriate. Later on seek out opportunities to make new friends.

8   Hope

Look to the future with optimism, and imagine how you would like your life to be. Focus on optimum healing.